A Contemporary Approach to Clinical Supervision

The most critical and influential relationship affecting one's growth as a mental health professional is the relationship between the clinician and the supervisor. Good supervisors breed good therapists. This book goes beyond facts and figures to provide an innovative perspective on the supervision process. Through contributions by seven supervisees and the supervisor they all shared, readers are offered a rare glimpse into what takes place during the supervision hour.

This book not only offers insight into the elements integral to effective supervision, but also teaches about the supervisory relationship. With contributors from various disciplines, theoretical orientations, and cultures, it shows how the supervisee and supervisor are able to navigate these differences while still gaining the most from supervision. Topics that are covered include cultural competence in multicultural supervision and remote supervision when it is conducted between clinicians in different countries, as well as an original study by the authors on the experiences of supervisees during the global Covid-19 pandemic and the transition to remote supervision.

For mental health professionals who are training to be supervisors or experienced supervisors looking to improve their skills, this book will serve as an invaluable resource for professional development.

Liat Shklarski is an assistant professor at Ramapo College of New Jersey School of Social Science and Human Services, Department of Social Work, and an adjunct professor at Smith College, School of Social Work. Her academic research focuses on effective clinical supervision. She is a graduate of the Contemporary Freudian Society psychodynamic psychotherapy training program and a licensed clinical social worker with a private psychotherapy practice. She works with individuals, couples, and youth with a history of trauma.

Allison Abrams is a licensed clinical social worker and psychotherapist practicing in New York City. She completed her postgraduate training at the Contemporary Freudian Society and the Psychoanalytic Association of New York, which is affiliated with NYU Medical School. She is an author and contributing writer for several publications, including *Psychology Today*, *GoodTherapy*, and *Verywell Mind*.

"In this collection of scholarly and stimulating essays. supervisees from a variety of cultural backgrounds describe conditions most conducive to learning. They also teach us the ways in which supervisions can go awry. Through clinical cases shared with a perceptive supervisor, we watch learning and teaching processes unfold. We are shown in detail just how complex and rewarding the supervisory experience can be."

Daniel Jacobs, MD, Training and Supervision Analyst, Boston Psychoanalytic Society and Institute, co-author, *The Supervisory Encounter*

"This book is distinctive, organized by two supervisees of an unusually gifted supervisor, written from supervisees' perspectives. It represents the insightful cumulation of the multiple supervisees' psychodynamic experiences. Readers will be delighted by their candid descriptions. The contributors demonstrate that supervision is the bilateral co-creative maturing process. It also delivers the implications of cross-cultural supervision. I guarantee that supervisees, supervisors, and many others in psychotherapy/psychoanalysis discipline will benefit significantly from reading this book world-wide."

Do-Un Jeong, MD, PhD, FIPA, Professor Emeritus, Seoul National University, Training/Supervising Analyst, IPA Korean Study Group

"This book is a wonderful tribute to the very special relationship that exists between supervisors and supervisees, encapsulating as it does the uniqueness and specialness of that relationship. I found myself immersed in this beautiful and unusual collection of essays, written by supervisees from diverse cultural and professional backgrounds. This is an important and compelling contribution to the literature on supervision. It will prove to be an invaluable asset to the field as well as an engaging read. If you want to become a better supervisor or gain more from supervision, then this book is for you."

Elise Snyder, MD, President of China American Psychoanalytic Alliance, Associate Clinical Professor, Yale School of Medicine

A Contemporary Approach to Clinical Supervision

The Supervisee Perspective

Edited by
Liat Shklarski and Allison Abrams

Routledge
Taylor & Francis Group
LONDON AND NEW YORK

First published 2021
by Routledge
2 Park Square, Milton Park, Abingdon, Oxon OX14 4RN

and by Routledge
605 Third Avenue, New York, NY 10158

Routledge is an imprint of the Taylor & Francis Group, an informa business

British Library Cataloguin-in-Publication Data
A catalogue record for this book is available from the British Library

Library of Congress Cataloging-in-Publication Data
A catalog record has been requested for this book

ISBN: 978-1-032-01879-9 (hbk)
ISBN: 978-1-032-01857-7 (pbk)
ISBN: 978-1-003-18088-3 (ebk)

Typeset in Times New Roman
by Taylor & Francis Books

Contents

Illustrations

Figures

Tables

Contributors

Allison Abrams, LCSW-R, is a licensed clinical social worker and psychotherapist practicing in New York City. She completed her postgraduate training at the Contemporary Freudian Society (CFS) and the Psychoanalytic Association of New York, which is affiliated with NYU Medical School. She is an author and contributing writer for several publications, including *Psychology Today, GoodTherapy*, and *Verywell Mind.*

Ally Barlow, LCSW, is a licensed clinical social worker with a background in community organizing. For over five years, she directed the family support team in an education-focused community-based organization in the South Bronx. Ally has previously worked with a variety of populations, including individuals living with HIV/AIDS and survivors of sex trafficking.

Moosuk Lee, MD, PhD, is a training and supervising analyst for the Korean Psychoanalytic Study Group of the International Psychoanalytic Association. Dr. Lee is a professor emeritus of Chonnam National University, South Korea, and a former president of the Korean Psychoanalytic Guest Study Group of the International Psychoanalytic Association (IPA).

Camille Maruccia-Lee, LCSW, is a training and supervising psychoanalyst at the Contemporary Freudian Society. She has been working as a psychoanalyst with adults and couples in private practice in Manhattan for more than 30 years.

Liat Shklarski, PhD, LCSW, is an assistant professor at Ramapo College of New Jersey School of Social Science and Human Services, Department of Social Work, and an adjunct professor at Smith College, School of Social Work. Her academic research focuses on effective clinical supervision. She is a graduate of the Contemporary Freudian Society psychodynamic psychotherapy training program and a licensed clinical social worker with a private psychotherapy practice. She works with individuals, couples, and youth with a history of trauma.

Barbara Stimmel, PhD, is a training and supervising analyst at the Contemporary Freudian Society (CFS) and the International Psychoanalytic Association (IPA). She is a past president of the CFS and a past associate secretary of the IPA. She is a member of the American Psychoanalytic Association (APSA) and a clinical assistant professor of psychiatry at Mount Sinai Medical Center. Dr. Stimmel was also the chair of the Committee on Psychoanalytic Education's (COPE) sub-committee on supervision for more than 10 years. In that capacity, she conducted an ongoing discussion group at the APSA's scientific meetings on supervision; and, with her committee, she created an online reading list of supervisory articles and initiated a continuing course on supervision at the APSA. Dr. Stimmel was the North American chair of the IPA Berlin Congress, and has published in major psychoanalytic journals.

Ruiqi Tian, MA, is a registered supervisor of the Chinese Psychological Society, a member of the China American Psychoanalytic Alliance, and an associate professor of psychology at the Psychological Research and Counseling Center at Southwest Jiaotong University in Chengdu, China. She is also in private practice, offering psychological consultation and supervision.

Foreword

Fred Busch

I once had the unforgettable experience of listening to four jazz musicians—who had never played with each other before—sit down for an impromptu session. Within a few minutes, and without any music in front of them, they were playing together. It was moving and also incomprehensible. How did these musicians who had only just met succeed in playing this complex jazz music so wonderfully? In talking with them afterward, I learned how each applied a mutual framework based on years of study, within which they were all intently *listening* to each other. I have come to see this as a model for supervision. We begin in a halting manner as we build toward a mutually shared framework and hopefully end where the two parties are listening to the multiple voices in the room, each adding their unique contribution, aiming to find something to learn and grow from.

I was reminded of this experience while reading this one-of-a-kind book in which professionals from diverse settings and with different levels of experience write about what it is like to be in supervision with Dr. Barbara Stimmel, a psychoanalyst in New York. Unlike the musicians I heard, who all played jazz, reading this group of supervisees' reports was like listening to a classical pianist, a folk musician, and a hip-hop artist all following the same conductor. What does it take to do this so well and to the satisfaction of this diverse group? Dr. Stimmel, an unabashed Freudian, does not tell us exactly—but her supervisees do.

The contributors' descriptions of Dr. Stimmel's supervision of a psychotherapist who reluctantly reveals that she uses CBT in her work with patients, her supervision of a psychiatrist in a psychoanalytic training program from a culture very different from her own, and her supervision of a social worker who runs an agency geared toward helping low-income families access much-needed resources uncover certain keys to ensuring the success of an effective supervisor–supervisee relationship. This book teaches us that a good supervisor should first and foremost be *open to learning*.

In describing her own journey in supervision, Dr. Stimmel first tells us how she approaches being a supervisor. In my own experience, becoming a supervisor at all levels is like learning to swim by being thrown in the water. Her approach is to preconsciously sift through her own supervisors' modes of working to start to find her path. In some situations, she is "all business"; in others, she hangs around a setting, waiting to see how she can be helpful and not offering ideas before there is another interested in them.

The supervisees in this book demonstrate that in more traditional supervision, a good supervisor can be tough, in the best sense. At a time when there seems to be an "anything goes" approach to psychotherapy and psychoanalysis, a good supervisor sets some non-negotiable standards that supervisees understand are there to benefit the patient and the therapist.

The profound collective voice of the supervisees of Dr. Stimmel demonstrates that an effective supervisor is able to let her supervisees know what she thinks of their work, which is something that many supervisors eschew because of their discomfort with saying anything that is not positive. I have heard many psychoanalysts say that they never heard anything about their method of working from their supervisors other than to say that they were doing "OK." Finally, I have the impression that all of the contributors to this book understood that Dr. Stimmel's goal in supervision was to help them grow in the direction they would like, rather than imposing her passionate interest and involvement in psychoanalysis on them.

In my own training, I have had few excellent supervisors. I wish Dr. Stimmel had been one of them. After reading this book, I think most people would feel the same.

Fred Busch
Chestnut Hill, MA

Preface

About a year ago, during a supervision session, I (Liat) began by telling my supervisor, Dr. Barbara Stimmel, that I had a "crazy" idea I wanted to share with her—but only if she promised not to laugh at me. At the time, I had just completed my doctorate, so I had some relatively "free" time on my hands. I wanted to write a book about my work as a psychotherapist—specifically about the concepts that I have learned and that I continue to apply in the work I do with almost all of my patients. These are concepts that I have learned from Barbara over the six years of supervision that I have had with her. I said, "Barbara, I want to write a book about you." Of course, she did not make fun of me at all; instead, she smiled and was quick to say that the book should not be about *her* but about *supervision*. At this point, I stopped listening—I was just excited that I had gotten Barbara's approval!

The journey continued that Friday evening after my meeting with Barbara. My best friend, Allison Abrams, whom I met while we were students at the Psychoanalytic Training Institute of the Contemporary Freudian Society (CFS) and who had recommended Barbara to me as a supervisor, came over for Shabbat dinner. My family and I love having her with us almost every Friday night; we enjoy the conversation, laughing, talking nonsense, politics, and making jokes.

That Friday was different. I almost jumped on Allison. "Want to write a book together?" I asked. Allison, always ready for an adventure, and trusting me, first said yes and then later asked what the book would be about. Shabbat dinner soon became a work meeting. With kids running around, both of us stuffed after a good meal and tired from the week, by the end of the night we had drafted what would later become our book proposal. From that point on, the journey was no longer my own, but ours.

* * *

I (Allison) was incredibly honored that night when Liat asked me to write this book with her. The idea of working on a project that would combine my two passions—psychotherapy and writing—sounded like a dream. That it would be a project on which I would collaborate with my best friend made it that much more special.

Liat explained that she wanted to write about our experiences in supervision with Barbara Stimmel and how they have influenced our professional lives and our growth as clinicians. This greatly resonated with me because Barbara has been such an influence on me as a supervisor—so much so that I had recommended Barbara to Liat when we were both training at the CFS. I had a feeling they would mesh, just as Barbara and I had. Needless to say, they did. Six years and hundreds of supervision sessions later, here we are. Venturing on the journey to write this book was one of the most memorable parts of that Friday night—second only to Liat's homemade chocolate cake. I can only hope that the ingredients we used to create this book have produced a work as satisfying and as delicious as that dessert!

Acknowledgments

There were innumerable people who supported us on this journey, helped shape our experiences and thinking, and provided us with implicit and explicit resources that made this work possible. We would like to express our special appreciation for Barbara Stimmel, who has been our mentor throughout this journey. She has taught us more than we could ever give her credit for here. Her support and encouragement have been critical, and we are so grateful.

We are truly thankful to the book's contributors, who invested their precious time in meeting with us, writing, and editing their chapters. Their contributions made this idea come to life. We also want to thank our colleague, Kitrina Bevan, whose contribution was invaluable to the success of this project.

Acknowledgments are all about thanking the people who were most significant to our professional development and the accomplishment of the book. During our supervision, we indirectly came to know a person whom we never had the opportunity to meet in person: Barry Stimmel. Barbara's husband, who passed away in November 2014, has been an integral part of our supervisory relationship with Barbara. He has often been present in the room through Barbara's stories about his special personality and their rich life together.

Our heartfelt thanks to our families for always being so supportive of our work. A special thanks to Allison's family, friends, teachers, colleagues, and mentors—specifically, to supervisors extraordinaire Dale Daley, Lynnell Herzer, Dr. Amy Vigliotti, and to Dr. Stephanie Jones, whose support along the journey has been invaluable. Thank you to Liat's husband, Gil, who has always had faith in our ability to make this happen, and has made this journey possible without complaint and with a lot of support. To Liat's children, Hilah, Eitan, and Yonatan, who agreed to watch unlimited TV while we worked on the book—thank you. And finally, to all of our patients, we extend our thanks.

Chapter 1

Defining effective supervision through the eyes of the supervisee

A contemporary systematic review

Liat Shklarski and Allison Abrams

Introduction

In this chapter, we will first explore the meaning of the term "clinical supervision"; then, we will focus on the definition of effective clinical supervision as it is described in the literature; and finally, we will report our findings based on a systematic review undertaken as part of the preparatory research for this book.

There is ample literature and research on clinical supervision in the field of mental health (e.g., psychology, social work, psychoanalytic training, etc.). However, research exploring effective supervision from the point of view of the supervisee is limited. In order to support our work with empirical knowledge, we conducted a systematic review of databases to locate the most recent empirical literature focusing on effective supervision from the perspective of supervisees. In particular, we were curious to find out more about (1) the experiences of supervisees in supervision; and (2) supervision outcomes based on supervisees' perceptions of the working alliance with their supervisor.

Overview of clinical supervision

The question "What is clinical supervision?" is a very complex one. It is almost impossible to answer because it depends on the profession, career stage, educational stage (undergraduate, graduate, or postgraduate), and discipline (e.g., social work, psychology, licensed mental health counseling, licensed marriage and family therapy, art therapy) of the supervisee, as well as the setting where the supervision takes place. A quick search for the keywords "clinical supervision" in a scholarly database yields results on supervision in the medical and helping professions, such as nursing, education, clinical psychology, and social work.

How do we define clinical supervision? Most definitions emphasize that clinical supervision is a form of relationship-based education and training that promotes professional development (Milne, 2009; Counseling Students & Pearson, 2004). Snowdon et al. (2015) define clinical supervision as a process that enhances growth and increases skills in supervisees who are working toward their own professional licensing requirements or are eager to improve their professional skills. During supervision, supervisees learn and refine the clinical skills needed to provide effective psychotherapy (Falender, 2018; Falender & Shafranske, 2014). The supervisor helps the supervisee make sense of the therapeutic work. This in turn becomes internalized by the supervisee and is pulled out whenever necessary (Aronson, 2000).

The roots of clinical supervision can be traced back to the late 1800s, when Sigmund Freud first engaged in peer consultations with Josef Breuer and provided psychodynamically oriented supervision to Max Graf on how best to help his emotionally troubled son, Little Hans (Fleming & Steen, 2013; Watkins, 2013). This type of supervision did not have a structured model and was based on letter exchanges and face-to-face meetings. Since then, supervision has become a routine aspect of good practice. More clinicians, managers, and supervisors understand that supervision is necessary to improve client care, develop the professionalism of clinical personnel, and impart and maintain ethical standards in the field. In fact, all formal clinical training—including in the fields of psychology, social work, mental health counseling, psychotherapy, and psychoanalysis—requires students to attend supervision to consult on cases and connect theory and practice. It is also important to remember that in other cases, particularly within organizations, clinical supervision has become the cornerstone of quality improvement and assurance, specifically when supervision is given in the workplace and at times combined with administrative supervision (Tromski-Klingshirn & Davis, 2007).

Effective supervision

What is the recipe for effective clinical supervision? Effective supervision has been connected to improved clinical and client outcomes and a positive impact on therapist self-awareness, skills, self-efficacy, theoretical orientation, and support (Egan et al., 2017; Wheeler & Richards, 2007). A common factor shown to be significantly tied to positive supervision outcomes is the concept of the supervisory working alliance (Ladany & Lehrman-Waterman, 1999; Lucas, 2018). Park et al. (2019) use Bordin's (1983) definition of the supervisory working alliance that consists of three interrelated variables: agreement on the goals of supervision, the tasks of supervision, and an emotional bond between the trainee and the supervisor. The supervisory working alliance fosters confidence, promotes exploration of countertransference, and improves supervisees' self-awareness and self-efficacy (Callahan & Love, 2020).

Supervisor–supervisee interactions can positively or negatively affect the supervisory working alliance. As a result, supervisors and supervisees must figure out their own authentic way of working together. Contrastano (2020) discussed reciprocal vulnerability in which the supervisor is willing to be vulnerable and uses self-disclosure as an educational tool. Reciprocal vulnerability deepens the relationship and improves the learning experience.

Following the notion that effective supervision relates to the quality of the supervisory relationship, Kilminster and Jolly (2000) conducted a literature review of 55 empirical studies on clinical supervision. They found a recurrent theme across all studies—that the relationship between supervisor and supervisee is a more significant determinant of supervision effectiveness than the supervisory methods that are used. A high association between effective supervision and a strong supervisory relationship is found with supervisors who are empathetic, supportive, respectful, and knowledgeable (Beinart & Clohessy, 2017; Callahan & Love, 2020; Lizzio et al., 2009). Ellis (2017) captured examples of negative supervision experiences including, but not limited to, boundary issues, dishonesty, disrespect, lack of supervisory competency, and/or perceived ethical misconduct/violations by supervisors that adversely affect the supervision process and supervisees' growth.

The supervisory working alliance can be compared to the therapeutic alliance (Enlow et al., 2019). For example, Watkins (2018) adapted and modified the generic model of psychotherapy developed by Orlinsky and Howard (1987) to create a generic model of psychotherapy supervision (GMPS) (see Figure 1.1). The organizational framework of the GMPS conceptualized the multiple variables that determine effective supervision. It enhanced understanding of the entire process of supervision, including mediating variables that can effectively influence the supervisory working alliance. The GMPS presents the complexity and interconnectedness of the input variables, supervision process, and output variables that affect the supervisory relationship. Both the supervisor and supervisee should be aware of these factors.

Input variables

The input variables are pre-existing features that include: (a) the supervisee's personal/professional/educational characteristics; (b) the supervisor's personal/professional/educational characteristics; (c) the community and organization in which supervision occurs; and (d) the social and cultural beliefs and values of the supervisor and supervisee.

Supervision process

The supervision process is the core of the model and consists of six critical components that are part of any supervisory relationship: the supervision contract, supervision operations, the supervision bond, self-relatedness (supervisee and supervisor), in-session impacts, and temporal patterns. In particular, the supervision process focuses on (a) all interactions that are experienced by the supervisor and supervisee during supervision sessions; and (b) any supervisor or supervisee experiences or actions that occur outside of supervision sessions (e.g., further reflections on the supervision session).

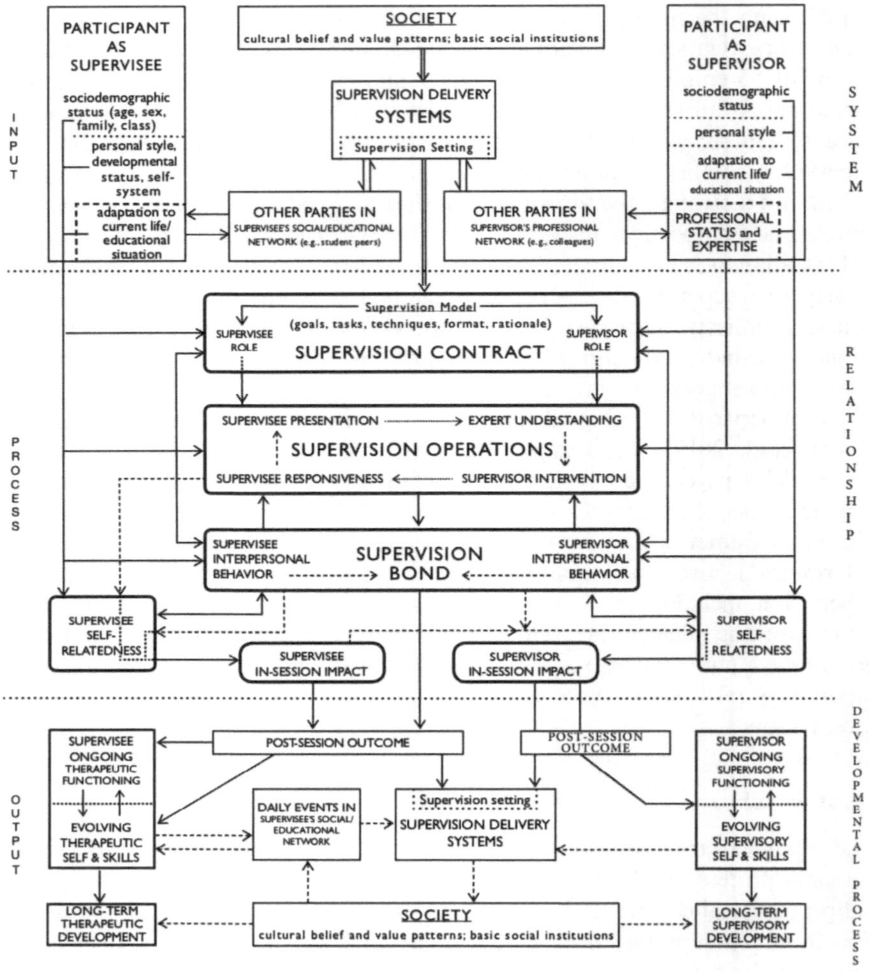

Figure 1.1 A generic model of psychotherapy supervision
Source: Watkins (2018). Reproduced with permission.

Output variables

Outputs are postsession supervision outcomes that occur in the real world for both the supervisees and their patients. Outputs contribute to the ongoing therapeutic functioning of the supervisee in their role as a therapist and the ongoing supervisory functioning of the supervisor (i.e., outputs contribute to their respective outside-session development).

The GMPS highlights that supervisory relationships are interrelated with many factors and require in-depth, holistic thinking. In order to add knowledge to the model, in particular the supervision process, we focus our systematic review on the supervision process from the supervisee's perspective.

Systematic review of the empirical literature on effective supervision from the supervisee's perspective

Despite the ample literature on supervision, few studies have been based on empirical research, and even fewer have been both empirical and captured the perspective of the supervisee. It is widely assumed by policy-makers, educators, and practitioners that supervision is a good thing. But does the available research, specifically that which expresses the voice of the supervisee, support this assumption about effective supervision?

Search strategy

We based our procedure for conducting and reporting a systematic review on the approaches documented by Stroup et al. (2000). Accordingly, we undertook an initial comprehensive electronic search of the literature. Boolean operations of supervisee AND (clinical supervision* OR supervision* supervisory relationship* OR analytic training* OR psychotherapy* OR parallel process) OR effective clinical supervision AND (supervisee perspective OR supervisees' perceptions OR supervisees' experiences) were used to identify relevant articles in the identified databases. The initial search was conducted in March 2020, with one additional search conducted in April 2020.

Databases

Databases were selected based on previous literature reviews on clinical supervision. EBSCOhost was used to search Academic Search Premier, CINAHL, Medline, PsychInfo, Professional Development Collection, Psychology and Behavioral Sciences Collection, Social Work Abstracts, and SocioIndex. Additionally, PubMed was searched for relevant articles. Psychoanalytic Electronic Publishing (PEP-Web) was used to search for psychoanalytic literature and research.

Within systematic reviews such as this one, judgments need to be made with regard to the relative quality of the study(ies) and the evidence produced. Accordingly, each of the 167 papers included in the full review were examined for and evaluated on the basis of the following inclusion criteria: quantitative, mixed-methods, or qualitative peer-reviewed studies available in full text and in English (see Table 1.1). Because clinical supervision is a global field, studies from countries outside of the United States were included as long as the results were available in English. Articles published from 2000 to 2020 were included in this review.

Table 1.1 Inclusion criteria

1. Quantitative, qualitative, or mixed-methods studies.
2. Available in full text through Smith College in English.
3. Must feature supervisees' experiences.
4. Peer-reviewed articles.
5. Disciplines: social work, psychology, licensed mental health counseling, psychoanalysis.
6. Must have been published between 2000 and 2020.

Search results

A total of 1420 studies were identified across the databases (see Figure 1.2). The results of the database searches were downloaded into Zotero version 4.0.20 and duplicates were removed, yielding 537 studies for preliminary review. Of the 537

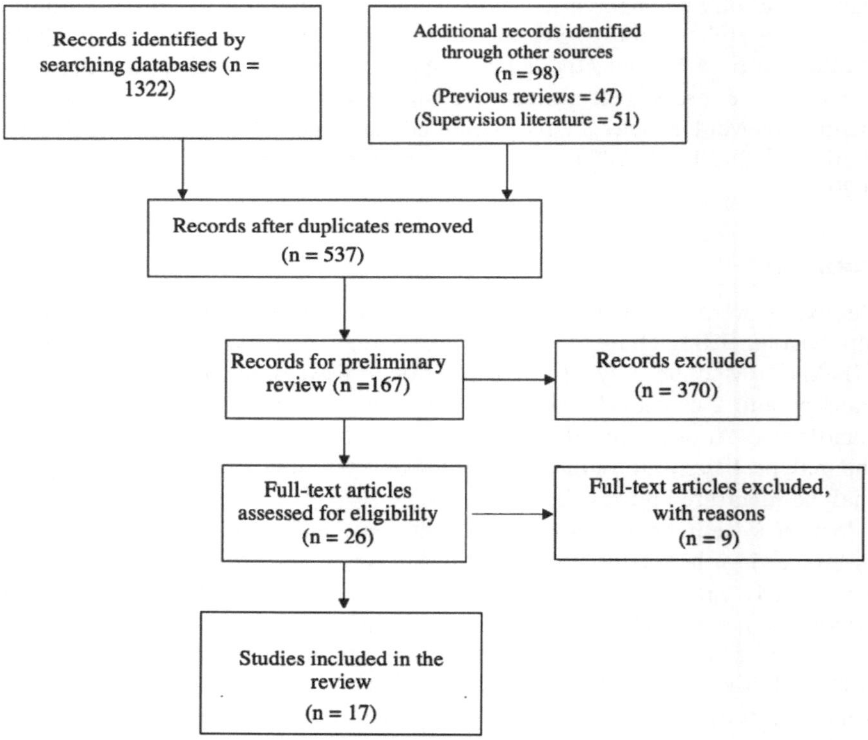

Figure 1.2 Search strategy

Table 1.2 Studies excluded after full-text review (n = 9)

Author (year)	*Reason for exclusion*
Ancis & Marshall (2010)	Supervisees' perceptions focused on cultural elements, which will be discussed in Chapter 2.
Bender & Dykeman (2016)	Topic focused on supervisees' perceptions of effective cyber supervision.
Callahan et al. (2019)	Method was excluded: the article presented a theoretical grounding and overview of the research on supervision.
Dawson et al. (2012)	Participants were from allied professions, meaning that only part of the sample was comprised of counselors, psychologists, or social workers.
Ellis (2017)	Method was not presented in the article.
Gardner et al. (2018)	Participants were from allied professions, meaning that only part of the sample was comprised of counselors, psychologists, or social workers.
Grassetti et al. (2019)	Supervisees' perceptions focused on motherhood and effective supervision.
Tromski-Klingshirn & Davis (2007)	Focused on supervisees' perspectives on effective supervision with supervisors who had a dual role of clinical and administrative supervisor.
West & Clark (2004)	Sample was too small: three supervisor–supervisee dyads.

studies reviewed for relevance based on their title and abstract content, 167 were eligible for full-text examination. Examination of the studies' text based on the inclusion criteria confirmed 17 applicable studies and 9 ineligible studies (Table 1.2 provides a list of the ineligible studies). The primary focus of this review was the analysis and synthesis of quantitative and qualitative articles focusing on clinical supervision from the perspective of the supervisee. However, many studies were eliminated because of a lack of clear methodology and multiple disciplines that did not fit the inclusion criteria.

Our process contained a number of steps. First, we identified and recorded whether the study produced qualitative, quantitative, or mixed-methods data. Second, we looked at whether the reported qualitative and quantitative findings were positive, negative, both, or neither in terms of the effects and impacts of clinical supervision. Last, we identified themes that captured all the findings and were representative of the body of evidence within the selected studies.

Overview of the studies

Table 1.3 provides an overview of the reviewed studies and details the aims of each study, their design, subject, samples, instrument measures, research findings,

Table 1.3 Data matrix of included studies

Author	*Method/ research design*	*Study aim*	*Target population/discipline*	*Significant findings*
Snowdon et al. (2015)	Quantitative instrument: Manchester Clinical Supervision Scale	To evaluate the effectiveness of the clinical supervision of psychotherapists.	60 registered psychotherapists.	More than half of the participants rated their supervision as less than effective. Participants found it difficult to find time for clinical supervision despite recognizing its value and importance.
Rousmaniere & Ellis (2013)	Quantitative instrument: Collaborative Supervision Behaviors Scale	To identify supervisees' perspectives on collaborative clinical supervision.	252 students from clinical psychology, school counseling, and clinical social work programs.	Effective supervision is dependent on collaboration between the supervisee and the supervisor. It requires the supervisee to be proactive.
Cook et al. (2018)	Quantitative instrument: Power Dynamics in Supervision Scale	To assess how supervisees perceive power dynamic issues in the supervisory relationship.	267 master's- and doctoral-level supervisees from counseling psychology, school psychology, and counselor education programs.	Supervisees perceived themselves as possessing the most power in terms of maintaining healthy boundaries with their supervisors and being willing to be vulnerable. Supervisees perceived their supervisors as possessing the most power when identifying which interventions to use with clients and providing feedback.

(*Continued*)

Table 1.3 (Cont.)

Author	*Method/ research design*	*Study aim*	*Target population/discipline*	*Significant findings*
Calvert et al. (2020)	Quantitative instrument: Metacommunication in Supervision Questionnaire	To identify the use of metacommunication in supervision from supervisees' perspectives and the nature of the supervisory relationship.	129 students and graduates of a psychology program receiving individual clinical supervision.	Various forms of metacommunication were used by supervisees, such as whether their needs were being met in supervision and negotiation of the terms of supervision. However, communication about uncomfortable feelings and negative evaluations was less common.
Pack (2012)	Qualitative instrument: In-depth interviews	To determine what clinical supervision means by comparing and contrasting the perspectives of clinical supervisors and their supervisees.	12 supervisees (social work and occupational therapy) and 10 clinical supervisors.	The term "clinical supervision" was understood differently by the supervisors and the supervisees. Supervisees emphasized supervision as a safe space with a trusting and supportive relationship, while supervisors emphasized supervision as a way of ensuring safe practice.
Murphy & Wright (2005)	Qualitative instrument: Semi-structured interviews	To identify supervisees' perceptions of the use of power by their clinical supervisors.	11 supervisees in a marriage and family therapy education training program.	Supervisees expected their supervisors to have and use power. They viewed the appropriate use of this power as contributing to their clinical growth. Empowerment and collaboration were seen as positive uses of power by supervisees.

(*Continued*)

Table 1.3 (Cont.)

Author	*Method/ research design*	*Study aim*	*Target population/discipline*	*Significant findings*
Green & Dekkers (2010)	Quantitative instrument: Online survey with 70 questions, including the Feminist Supervision Scale and a supervision feedback form	To assess the perspectives of supervisees on the attention given to power and diversity in supervision in relation to satisfaction and learning outcomes.	42 supervisees and 22 supervisors from accredited marriage and family therapy programs.	Supervisees were more satisfied with supervision when the supervisor utilized feminist practices (e.g., collaborative relationship, power analysis, diversity and social context, and advocacy).
Gazzola & Theriault (2007)	Qualitative instrument: Semi-structured interviews	To assess the perspectives of supervisees on broadening (effective) and narrowing (ineffective) experiences in supervision.	10 supervisees in a counseling master's degree program.	Narrowing experiences included a lack of supervisor flexibility, inadequate feedback, a dysfunctional relationship dynamic, and a lack of sensitivity. Broadening experiences included validation and empowerment, a nurturing environment to promote professional growth, and positive personal qualities (positive energy).
O'Donoghue (2012)	Qualitative instrument: Semi-structured interviews	To understand how social workers develop their understanding, participation, and use of supervision based on their past and present experiences in supervision.	16 social workers who were in supervision at the time of the study.	Participants reported that having an external supervisor (outside of the workplace) was effective. Participants who had significant previous experiences in supervision were aware of their needs in supervision.

(*Continued*)

Table 1.3 (Cont.)

Author	*Method/ research design*	*Study aim*	*Target population/discipline*	*Significant findings*
Anderson et al. (2000)	Quantitative instrument: Survey developed for the purposes of the study	To identify supervisees' perceptions of their best and worst supervision experiences.	98 students in marriage and family therapy education training programs.	The frequency of supervision and consistency were associated with positive experiences, as was providing feedback in a straightforward manner and encouraging experimentation. Poor experiences included indirect and avoidant communication and supervisors' preoccupations with their own problems.
Shaffer & Friedlander (2017)	Quantitative instruments: 1 Relational Behavior Scale (RBS) 2 Working Alliance Inventory-Trainee 3 Trainee Personal Reaction Scale-Revised	To assess the association between strong alliance perceptions and positive evaluations of the supervisor.	141 trainees in counseling and clinical psychology doctoral programs and master's programs in mental health counseling, social work, and couples and family therapy.	Relational behavior of the supervisor is associated with a positive supervisory alliance. A strong alliance contributes to trainees' positive experiences of their supervisors.

(*Continued*)

Table 1.3 (Cont.)

Author	*Method/ research design*	*Study aim*	*Target population/discipline*	*Significant findings*
Lizzio et al. (2009)	Quantitative instrument: 1 Supervisor Relating Style Inventory 2 Self-reported five-item scale about supervision effectiveness	To identify supervisees' perceptions of the impact of relationship dimensions (e.g., supervisor support, challenges, and openness) on supervisee anxiety and the perceived effectiveness of supervision.	261 psychology graduates actively in supervision.	Supervisees' perceptions of supervisor support and openness predicted supervisor effectiveness. Positive influences through the relationship process reduced supervisees' self-reported levels of defensiveness in the supervisory process.
Nelson & Friedlander (2001)	Mixed-methods instrument: 1 Supervisory Styles Inventory 2 Role Conflict and Ambiguity Inventory 3 Semi-structured interviews	To identify the perspectives of supervisees on negative experiences in supervision.	13 master's and doctoral trainees in psychology.	Power struggles and dual relationships were associated with negative experiences in supervision.
Daniel et al. (2015)	Quantitative instrument: A three-item self-reported questionnaire (mindfulness, supervisory relationship, and session dynamics)	To identify supervisors' and supervisees' self-ratings of mindfulness, predicted perceptions of the supervisory relationship, and session dynamics.	144 participants: 72 pairs of supervisors and supervisees from counseling and related educational programs.	Supervisors' self-ratings of mindfulness were predictive of the supervision variables but supervisees' self-ratings of mindfulness were not.

(*Continued*)

Table 1.3 (Cont.)

Author	*Method/ research design*	*Study aim*	*Target population/discipline*	*Significant findings*
Fernando & Hulse-Killacky (2005)	Quantitative instrument: 1 Supervisory Styles Inventory 2 Supervisory Satisfaction Questionnaire 3 Counseling Self-Estimate Inventory	To identify supervisees' perceptions of supervisors' supervisory styles (attractive, interpersonally sensitive, task-oriented) and their satisfaction with supervision.	82 counseling students from six master's-level counselor education programs.	Effective supervision was correlated with all three supervisory styles. However, interpersonally sensitive was the most effective of the three.
Knox et al. (2014)	Qualitative instrument: Semi-structured interviews	To identify supervisees' perceptions of the internal representations of their clinical supervisors and their connection to the supervisory relationship.	11 doctoral students from clinical psychology and counseling psychology programs.	A positive internal representation of the supervisor was associated with a strong working alliance.
Egan et al. (2017)	Mixed-methods instrument: 1 Open-ended questions in an online survey 2 Focus groups including health/counseling practice professionals	To identify supervisees' perspectives on effective supervisory relationships.	237 social work supervisees.	A safe supervisory environment was associated with effective supervision. Effective supervision within organizations was jeopardized by the dual role of the supervisor (as a manager and a supervisor).

limitations, and quality of evidence rating. Based on our review, we grouped the data into four categories related to effective supervision: (1) balancing power dynamics between the supervisor and supervisee; (2) a safe and nurturing space; (3) supervisee's commitment to the supervisory relationship, and; (4) pedagogical viewpoint and professional experience of the supervisor.

Balancing power dynamics between the supervisor and supervisee

Supervisors hold more of the power in the supervisory relationship, and it is therefore important that they are aware of it. The extent to which power is exercised within the supervisory work impacts the supervisee's learning experiences and ability to grow professionally. In our review, some of the studies (n = 5) addressed power dynamics as a common factor influencing effective supervision. Cook et al. (2018) used the Power Dynamics in Supervision Scale (PDSS) to assess supervisees' perceptions of power dynamics in supervision by using a feminist conceptual framework that challenges the power given to the supervisor and encourages the process to be equal between the supervisor and the supervisee. Supervision was perceived as highly effective when the supervisee reported that they had a degree of power and that their supervisor used their power positively. In this study, 267 supervisees from counseling psychology programs filled out the PDSS. The results showed that effective supervision was associated with a supervisee's ability to maintain healthy boundaries, feel vulnerable in supervision, and feel empowered in supervision. As for their supervisors, the participants perceived supervision to be effective when their supervisors demonstrated their power by identifying interventions to use with patients and providing constructive feedback, as well as treating supervisees like colleagues when discussing clinical cases (Cook et al., 2018).

Similar results were reported by Green and Dekkers (2010), whose findings emphasized supervisees' expectations that their supervisors would address diversity and power in the supervisory relationship. They conducted a quantitative study using the Feminist Supervision Scale with 42 supervisees from marriage and family therapy programs and 22 supervisors. They found that when supervisors were competent in addressing issues of diversity and power, supervisees reported a higher level of satisfaction with their supervisors.[1] Supervisees reported higher levels of satisfaction with supervisors who addressed these issues, while supervisors did not perceive them as influencing the quality of the supervisory relationship.

While the Green and Dekkers study results on power dynamics seem to be ideal, Calvert et al. (2020) reported a different reality. One hundred and twenty-nine clinical psychologists participated in their survey on the supervisory relationship focusing on supervisor communication. The findings from this study showed that at times participants hesitated to directly communicate about adverse events, disagreements, or discomfort with their supervisors, and their expressions of discomfort/vulnerability did not occur often. Participants were hesitant to bring up disagreements or concerns around negative evaluations from their supervisors.

A positive outlook from the Calvert et al. study showed that the number of years in supervision had a positive correlation with supervisees' ability to discuss adverse events. In other words, long-term supervisory relationships create safer spaces in which to discuss challenges in the supervisory relationship. This notion is supported by several studies (Anderson et al., 2000; O'Donoghue, 2012). For example, the best supervision experiences were associated with a significantly longer duration and included discussions of a greater number of cases.

Nelson and Friedlander (2001) captured the negative experiences of supervisory relationships with a sample of 13 counseling psychology trainees. They used the Supervisory Styles Inventory and semi-structured interviews to assess the factors that have a negative impact on supervisees' experiences in supervision. For example, supervisees who felt that their supervisors reacted with anger or were too busy for them reported that they were deeply hurt and less invested in the supervisory relationship as a result. Participants also highlighted that some supervisors were not willing to own their role in the conflict, and constantly engaged in an unhealthy power dynamic. While this study used a very small sample, it is important to highlight how ineffective supervision and supervisors' lack of awareness can harm their supervisees' professional competencies and confidence.

Daniel et al. (2015) quantitatively surveyed 72 pairs of supervisors and supervisees (n = 144) regarding the supervisors' ability to be mindful and to pay attention in a non-judgmental way. The results from the dyadic data support previous findings: participants perceived supervisors who demonstrated mindfulness during their supervision work and paid attention to the supervisee's individual needs as better supervisors. They found that having greater alignment on supervisory goals and tasks was associated with a deeper and more powerful supervisory relationship.

A safe and nurturing space

Effective supervision is based on the relationship between the supervisor and the supervisee and not only on the clinical or the psychodynamic model of clinical supervision. In particular, effective supervision is associated with finding a balance between feeling supported and challenged to venture outside of one's comfort zone. Some studies (n = 8), the majority of which were qualitative, highlighted that effective supervision relates to the supervisee's ability to feel safe, empowered, and respected. For example, Pack (2012) interviewed eight social work supervisees and their supervisors. In that study, the participants reported that the quality of the supervision was dependent on supervisees feeling that the relationship was safe and that there was mutual respect, no judgment, and a consistent and continuous two-way dialogue. Participants linked effective supervision to the supervisor's feedback; they expected their supervisors to strike a balance between offering a critique (e.g., helping the supervisee to develop their own style of work) and providing positive reinforcement (e.g., confirming that they were on the right track).

Following this example, Egan et al. (2017) conducted a mixed-methods study with 476 social workers. Participants filled out a survey about trust, power, and safety in their supervisory relationship, and about 10 percent of the participants participated in a focus group. The findings from this study highlighted the strong connection between trustful relationships and professional growth, noting that "challenging elements occur when a supervisor knows how to challenge in an appropriate and safe way" (Egan et al., 2017, p. 314). Participants reported that having a trustful relationship with a supervisor resulted in a less stressful dynamic and increased their confidence. In this study, the participants described the safe space as a tool for professional development. Through critical self-reflection that involved reciprocity, they were able to develop their clinical skills.

Murphy and Wright (2005) qualitatively studied the perceptions of 11 supervisees in marriage and family therapy training on power dynamics in the supervisory relationship. Consistent with other studies, the authors found that promoting an atmosphere of safety and empowerment helped to form an effective supervisory relationship. A positive use of power was perceived by supervisees as the supervisor's ability to provide sometimes uncomfortable feedback in a way that fostered clinical growth, to appropriately self-disclose professional and personal information, and to be trustworthy and flexible when needed.

Similar findings were found in a quantitative study by Lizzio et al. (2009). They found that effective supervision was associated with supervisors who provided positive feedback and emphasized positive work. It was important for supervisees to feel that their supervisors recognized their strengths and abilities. The participants in that study reported feeling less anxious or defensive when their supervisors approached challenges with positivity.

A safe supervisory relationship is also important because it may impact supervisees' self-efficacy and confidence. Fernando and Hulse-Killacky (2005) assessed the relation between supervisory styles and satisfaction with supervision using the Supervisory Styles Inventory with 82 students pursuing a master's degree in counseling. The findings showed that attractive styles ("friendly," "trusting," and "supportive") and interpersonally sensitive styles ("intuitive," "invested," and "reflective") were associated with high satisfaction with the supervisory relationship. A task-oriented style ("structured," "evaluative," and "goal-oriented" supervision) was associated with a lower level of satisfaction and lower level of perceived self-efficacy among supervisees.

In order for supervisees to be challenged and pushed beyond their comfort level, supervisors must create a safe atmosphere. Gazzola and Theriault (2007) qualitatively studied the positive and negative factors associated with effective supervision using ten graduates of a counseling program. Participants reported high levels of satisfaction with the supervisory relationship when their supervisors tailored their supervision to the supervisees' unique needs. They felt positive about supervision when their supervisors fostered an environment in which they could be vulnerable, creative, and think independently.

Anderson et al. (2000) found similar findings. They surveyed 160 marriage and family counselors about their positive and negative supervision experiences. The factors positively correlated with effective supervision included supervisors who demonstrated more interpersonal traits such as being friendly, likable, and warm. In addition, supervisors who provided feedback in a straightforward manner, were open to accepting feedback, and encouraged experimentation were perceived by supervisees as effective supervisors.

Shaffer and Friedlander (2017) explored different relational supervision strategies among 141 trainees in counseling and clinical psychology. In this study, the authors used the Relational Behavior Scale and the Working Alliance Inventory Trainee Scale. The results showed that participants found their supervisors' relational behavior to be effective and to improve their learning experiences. For example, supervisors who encouraged their supervisees to explore their feelings were found to be more effective.

Supervisee's commitment to the supervisory relationship

One would think that effective supervision is dependent on the degree of knowledge, expertise, and experience of the supervisor. Nevertheless, some studies (n = 4) have shown that effective supervision depends on the commitment of the supervisee to supervision and their sense of responsibility in preparing for meetings with the supervisor, taking notes, and implementing relevant materials in their clinical work. For instance, Snowdon et al. (2015) found that participants who perceived clinical supervision as important regardless of heavy workloads, busy schedules, and other barriers reported that the supervisory relationship was effective and influential in their professional development. This study was the only study that used the Manchester Clinical Supervision Scale, which is a scale designed to explore the perceived quality and effectiveness of clinical supervision from the supervisee's perspective. This finding is supported by a study done by Rousmaniere and Ellis (2013) on collaboration in clinical supervision and its effect on the quality of supervision. They used the Supervisory Working Alliance Inventory (trainee version) and the Collaborative Supervision Behavior Scale with 252 graduates of clinical psychology, social work, and counseling programs. They found that effective supervision is dependent on the supervisee's behaviors, proactiveness, and collaboration with the supervisor (such as through discussions about expectations, activities in supervision, and the working frame).

O'Donoghue (2012) interviewed 16 social workers about their past and present experiences in supervision, finding that participants who had positive supervisory relationships throughout their educational journeys were more likely to feel comfortable with their next supervisor. Supervisees' experiences were influenced by their commitment to the supervisory relationship, their active participation in the relationship, their investment in professional development, and their motivation to "grow" as clinicians. This study emphasized that ownership, proactivity, and the motivation of supervisees increased the effectiveness of supervision. Further, O'Donoghue found that positive supervision was associated with personalizing the supervisory relationship by working out a frame that fit the clinical needs of the supervisees.

The work of Daniel et al. (2015) on mindfulness in supervision also found the supervisee's commitment to the supervisory relationship to be important. While the authors highlighted the correlation between the supervisor's ability to be mindful and effective supervision, they also found connections between the supervisee's degree of mindfulness, attention to differences, and their ability to speak up in order to improve the working alliance.

Pedagogical viewpoint and professional experience of the supervisor

Some studies (n = 5) made a connection between effective supervision and the clinical expertise of the supervisor and their ability to contribute novel and exciting perspectives. Pack (2012) also found that supervisees expected their supervisors to have clinical experience, knowledge of theoretical approaches, and seniority within the clinical field. Similar findings were reported by Murphy and Wright (2005), who found that the best supervisory experience was associated with but not exclusive to the supervisor's expertise. O'Donoghue (2012) found that effective supervision was associated with supervisors who provided practical wisdom to assist supervisees in constructing and conceptualizing supervision. Similar findings showed that better experiences in supervision were associated with supervisees perceiving their supervisors as experts (Anderson et al., 2000).

It is important that supervisors do not impose their clinical orientation on their supervisees. Gazzola and Theriault (2007) reported that while supervisors' expertise was a very important component in effective supervision, negative experiences in supervision were associated with supervisors' rigid adherence to their own theoretical orientations. A lack of clinical flexibility or an invitation to participate in conceptualizing their cases provoked anxiety among supervisees. Shaffer and Friedlander (2017) suggested looking at relational supervision strategies. They found that effective supervision was associated with supervisors who focused on the therapeutic process (of the supervisees and their patients) and attended to the parallel process and countertransference. Lizzio et al.'s findings were similar. They surveyed 261 psychology graduates about the quality of their supervisory relationships. The participants reported that effective supervision was associated with how much their supervisor challenged them. They perceived supervision to be more effective when their supervisor invited them to examine their blind spots and challenged their assumptions or preconceived ideas. In addition, the researchers found that the supervisees experienced effective supervision when their supervisors openly discussed their own professional mistakes and made an effort to listen and understand, even when they strongly disagreed with their supervisee.

Finally, a different approach to understanding the connection between the knowledge of the supervisor and effective supervision was indirectly described in a study with 11 supervisees from clinical psychology programs. In that study, positive internal representations of supervisors were associated with a significant impact on the participants' professional development (Knox et al., 2014). For some of the participants, internal representations of their supervisor occurred when they experienced a difficult clinical moment that resulted in them thinking about their supervisor's possible reaction and reacting accordingly.

Discussion

Our systematic review of the existing empirical knowledge captured supervisees' perspectives on the factors that are associated with effective supervision. The four main categories of our review highlight that supervisors and supervisees are equally important players in forging a successful working alliance. The results of this study are supported by previous research that was done on the topic of effective supervision from the supervisee's perspective, particularly the work of Wilson et al. (2016), who conducted a systematic search of trainee therapists' supervision experiences. It is comforting to know that there is an ongoing effort to learn from supervisees in order to improve the supervisory working alliance.

Our findings showed that the supervisor and the supervisee share the goal of identifying opportunities to make use of power in a way that improves the supervisory relationship and builds a positive working alliance. It is important for both sides to be aware of their power and learn how to use it in a transparent way. For example, the supervisor can develop opportunities to engage in an open dialogue about possible conflicts or disagreements that might come up in the relationship and can be solved by conversation.

Another important factor predicting effective supervision is its ability to be a safe space for the supervisee. Our findings highlighted the importance of fostering a trustful relationship in which the supervisee can openly discuss their professional and personal vulnerabilities and in return receive constructive feedback. Our review aligns with previous research that showed how a "holding" environment in supervision leads to effective supervision.

The lines between supervision and therapy can become blurred, either by the novice supervisee or even inadvertently by the most seasoned supervisor. We believe that there should be a balance in supervision between the "professional" and the "personal." However, at times, the effective, safe, and nurturing space in supervision can unintentionally become a therapeutic space and damage the working alliance as a result. We recommend developing research that focuses on supervisees' perspectives on effective supervision in relation to personal self-disclosure.

One of the interesting findings of this review (which did not get enough attention in the literature) was the relationship between effective supervision and supervisees' commitment to supervision. We usually attribute successful supervision to the supervisor and the supervisor's knowledge; but some of the studies we reviewed highlighted the supervisee's commitment in terms of their preparation before supervisory meetings, their participation in meetings (such as by taking notes, asking questions, and engaging in roleplay), and their actions outside of supervision (such as their investment in implementing ideas with their patients) as being important factors influencing effective supervision.

Our findings show that the pedagogical viewpoint and the professional experience of the supervisor are linked to effective supervision; but the majority of the studies that we reviewed focused on the relational aspect of the supervision and less on the clinical experience of the supervisor. This is a very important factor that explains why supervision exists in the first place—to foster the ability to teach and the opportunity to learn. We recommend learning more about how supervisees perceive the level of knowledge of their supervisors and its influence on effective supervision.

From the little that we know, it is important to have a knowledgeable supervisor who has not only clinical experience but also the ability to teach and explain theory and practice. Similar to the supervisee's commitment to supervision, the professional experience of the supervisor is not particularly well covered by the research. This may be because in some cases, particularly in training programs, the supervisor is chosen by the institute and not by the future supervisee.

Limitations

While our review used strict inclusion criteria, we did not look at mediating variables to understand effective supervision. As a result, the findings covered all types of clinical supervisees' experiences and overlooked the unique experiences that supervisees in individual disciplines may have had. For example, do clinical psychologist trainees perceive effective supervision differently than students training to be mental health counselors, social workers, or family therapists? In addition, the studies we reviewed did not always specify the time frame of the supervision (i.e., how long the participants had been in a relationship with their supervisor), which may also have a significant influence on supervisees' perceptions of effective supervision.

Nor did the studies included in the review specify the cultural background of the participants or their supervisors. We wonder if effective supervision should also be understood through the lens of the cultural differences that exist between some supervisees and supervisors. This is a topic that we will explore in Chapter 3.

Future research

The lessons learned from this review can help foster a constructive and rewarding supervisory experience for both supervisors and supervisees. We believe that more research should be done to provide insight into the connection between effective supervision and supervisees' commitment to the supervisory working alliance. Next, we would like to learn more about the connection between effective supervision and the degree of supervisees' self-disclosure of personal details in supervision, a phenomenon that may occur once the relationship develops. But does the supervisor know where to draw the line between professional supervision and therapy while still maintaining a safe and nurturing space where supervisees feel comfortable with engaging in some self-disclosure? We also recommend investigating how supervisees choose their supervisors. Are certain components more important than others when choosing a supervisor?

It may also be beneficial to categorize supervisees' experiences according to their career stages. Our review showed that junior clinicians who were still in training had a harder time exercising their power in supervision. We are curious to know what effective supervision looks like with mature clinicians who are using supervision voluntarily (i.e., not as a training requirement).

Furthermore, we recommend investigating mediating variables that may influence supervision outcomes (e.g., the format of supervision, the educational background of the supervisor and the supervisee, payment, etc.). Such information could be helpful for both new supervisees with little experience in supervision and those who have experience in supervision. In addition, throughout our review, we noticed that many studies used various types of scales and inventories to assess effective supervision. Nevertheless, some of those tools were not assessed for their validity and reliability. It is recommended that researchers conduct studies about effective supervision utilizing valid and reliable instruments, such as the Working Alliance Inventory Trainee Scale (Palomo et al., 2010).

Finally, our review only included one-on-one supervision and did not cover effective group supervision. We recommend replicating this systematic review to learn about effective group supervision, mainly because many training institutes require supervisees to take part in group supervision. This is also true for clinicians who are already working and looking for more financially feasible supervision options, which group supervision offers.

Conclusions

If the number of studies and papers that focus on clinical supervision found in the current literature is any indication, there has recently been a gradual increase in the number of therapists/clinicians engaging in clinical supervision. Nevertheless, meaningful outcomes from supervisees' perspectives of effective supervision are lacking empirical evidence. The results of this review have implications for supervisees, supervisors, and researchers who can improve the supervisory working alliance and learn about how to provide effective supervision. Learning more about supervisees' perspectives on effective supervision can lead to new research on ways of choosing a supervisor and the factors related to sustaining a positive supervisory relationship. This chapter did not cover all of the possible mediating variables, but many will be examined in the following chapters, such as cultural diversity (Chapters 3, 4, and 5) and remote supervision (Chapters 2 and 5). We will also include the results of our innovative study looking at the effects of the Covid-19 pandemic and the subsequent transition to remote learning on the quality of supervision and the supervisory relationship (Chapter 2).

Note

1 Effective supervision with culturally diverse supervisees/supervisors will be further explored in Chapter 3.

References

Ancis, J. R., & Marshall, D. S. (2010). Using a multicultural framework to assess supervisees' perceptions of culturally competent supervision. *Journal of Counseling & Development*, 88(3), 277–284.

Anderson, S. A., Schlossberg, M., & Rigazio-DiGilio, S. (2000). Family therapy trainees' evaluations of their best and worst supervision experiences. *Journal of Marital and Family Therapy*, 26(1), 79–91.

Aronson, S. (2000). Analytic supervision: All work and no play? *Contemporary Psychoanalysis*, 36(1), 121–132.

Beinart, H., & Clohessy, S. (2017). *Effective supervisory relationships: Best evidence and practice.* Wiley.

Bender, S., & Dykeman, C. (2016). Supervisees' perceptions of effective supervision: A comparison of fully synchronous cybersupervision to traditional methods. *Journal of Technology in Human Services*, 34(4), 326–337.

Bordin, E. S. (1983). A working alliance based model of supervision. *The Counseling Psychologist*, 11(1), 35–42.

Callahan, J. L., & Love, P. K. (2020). Introduction to the special issue: Supervisee perspectives of supervision processes. *Journal of Psychotherapy Integration*, 30(1), 1–8. doi:10.1037/int0000199.

Callahan, J. L., Love, P. K., & Watkins, C. E., Jr. (2019). Supervisee perspectives on supervision processes: An introduction to the special issue. *Training and Education in Professional Psychology*, 13(3), 153–159. doi:10.1037/tep0000275.

Calvert, F. L., Deane, F. P., & Grenyer, B. F. (2020). Supervisee perceptions of the use of metacommunication in the supervisory relationship. *Psychotherapy Research*, 30 (2), 228–238.

Contrastano, C. M. (2020). Trainee's perspective of reciprocal vulnerability and boundaries in supervision. *Journal of Psychotherapy Integration*, 30(1), 44–51.

Cook, R. M., McKibben, W. B., & Wind, S. A. (2018). Supervisee perception of power in clinical supervision: The Power Dynamics in Supervision Scale. *Training and Education in Professional Psychology*, 12(3), 188–195.

Counseling Students, & Pearson, Q. M. (2004). Getting the most out of clinical supervision: Strategies for mental health. *Journal of Mental Health Counseling*, 26 (4), 361–373.

Daniel, L., Borders, L. D., & Willse, J. (2015). The role of supervisors' and supervisees' mindfulness in clinical supervision. *Counselor Education and Supervision*, 54 (3), 221–232.

Dawson, M., Phillips, B., & Leggat, S. G. (2012). Effective clinical supervision for regional allied health professionals: The supervisee's perspective. *Australian Health Review*, 36(1), 92–97.

Egan, R., Maidment, J., & Connolly, M. (2017). Trust, power and safety in the social work supervisory relationship: Results from Australian research. *Journal of Social Work Practice*, 31(3), 307–321.

Ellis, M. V. (2017). Narratives of harmful clinical supervision. *The Clinical Supervisor*, 36(1), 20–87.

Enlow, P. T., McWhorter, L. G., Genuario, K., & Davis, A. (2019). Supervisor–supervisee interactions: The importance of the supervisory working alliance. *Training and Education in Professional Psychology*, 13(3), 206–211.

Falender, C. A. (2018). Clinical supervision: The missing ingredient. *American Psychologist*, 73(9), 1240–1250.

Falender, C. A., & Shafranske, E. P. (2014). Clinical supervision: The state of the art. *Journal of Clinical Psychology*, 70(11), 1030–1041.

Fernando, D. M., & Hulse-Killacky, D. (2005). The relationship of supervisory styles to satisfaction with supervision and the perceived self-efficacy of master's-level counseling students. *Counselor Education and Supervision*, 44(4), 293–304.

Fleming, I., & Steen, L. (Eds.). (2013). *Supervision and clinical psychology: Theory, practice and perspectives*. Routledge.

Gardner, M. J., McKinstry, C., & Perrin, B. (2018). Effectiveness of allied health clinical supervision a cross-sectional survey of supervisees. *Journal of Allied Health*, 47 (2), 126–132.

Gazzola, N., & Theriault, A. (2007). Super- (and not-so-super-) vision of counsellors-in-training: Supervisee perspectives on broadening and narrowing processes. *British Journal of Guidance & Counselling*, 35(2), 189–204.

Grassetti, S. N., Pereira, L. M., Hernandez, E., & Fritzges-White, J. (2019). Conquering the maternal wall: Trainee perspectives on supervisory behaviors that assist in managing the challenges of new parenthood during clinical internship. *Training and Education in Professional Psychology*, 13(3), 200–205.

Green, M. S., & Dekkers, T. D. (2010). Attending to power and diversity in supervision: An exploration of supervisee learning outcomes and satisfaction with supervision. *Journal of Feminist Family Therapy*, 22(4), 293–312.

Kilminster, S. M., & Jolly, B. C. (2000). Effective supervision in clinical practice settings: A literature review. *Medical Education*, 34(10), 827–840.

Knox, S., Caperton, W., Phelps, D., & Pruitt, N. (2014). A qualitative study of supervisees' internal representations of supervisors. *Counselling Psychology Quarterly*, 27 (4), 334–352.

Ladany, N., & Lehrman-Waterman, D. E. (1999). The content and frequency of supervisor self-disclosures and their relationship to supervisor style and the supervisory working alliance. *Counselor Education and Supervision*, 38(3), 143–160.

Lizzio, A., Wilson, K., & Que, J. (2009). Relationship dimensions in the professional supervision of psychology graduates: Supervisee perceptions of processes and outcome. *Studies in Continuing Education*, 31(2), 127–140.

Lucas, K. M. (2018). *Understanding supervisee's experiences in clinical supervision from an attachment perspective.* [Unpublished doctoral dissertation]. University of Northern Colorado. https://digscholarship.unco.edu/dissertations/517.

Milne, D. (2009). *Evidence-based clinical supervision: Principles and practice.* Blackwell and British Psychological Society.

Murphy, M. J., & Wright, D. W. (2005). Supervisees' perspectives of power use in supervision. *Journal of Marital and Family Therapy*, 31(3), 283–295.

Nelson, M. L., & Friedlander, M. L. (2001). A close look at conflictual supervisory relationships: The trainee's perspective. *Journal of Counseling Psychology*, 48(4), 384–395. doi:10.1037/0022-0167.48.4.384.

O'Donoghue, K. (2012). Windows on the supervisee experience: An exploration of supervisees' supervision histories. *Australian Social Work*, 65(2), 214–231.

Orlinsky, D. E., & Howard, K. I. (1987). A generic model of psychotherapy. *Journal of Integrative & Eclectic Psychotherapy*, 6, 6–27.

Pack, M. (2012). Two sides to every story: A phenomenological exploration of the meanings of clinical supervision from supervisee and supervisor perspectives. *Journal of Social Work Practice*, 26(2), 163–179.

Palomo, M., Beinart, H., & Cooper, M. J. (2010). Development and validation of the Supervisory Relationship Questionnaire (SRQ) in UK trainee clinical psychologists. *British Journal of Clinical Psychology*, 49(2), 131–149.

Park, E. H., Ha, G., Lee, S., Lee, Y. Y., & Lee, S. M. (2019). Relationship between the supervisory working alliance and outcomes: A meta-analysis. *Journal of Counseling & Development*, 97(4), 437–446.

Rousmaniere, T. G., & Ellis, M. V. (2013). Developing the construct and measure of collaborative clinical supervision: The supervisee's perspective. *Training and Education in Professional Psychology*, 7(4), 300–308.

Shaffer, K. S., & Friedlander, M. L. (2017). What do "interpersonally sensitive" supervisors do and how do supervisees experience a relational approach to supervision? *Psychotherapy Research*, 27(2), 167–178.

Snowdon, D. A., Millard, G., & Taylor, N. F. (2015). Effectiveness of clinical supervision of physiotherapists: A survey. *Australian Health Review*, 39(2), 190–196.

Stroup, D. F., Berlin, J. A., Morton, S. C., Olkin, I., Williamson, G. D., Rennie, D., … & Thacker, S. B. (2000). Meta-analysis of observational studies in epidemiology: A proposal for reporting. *Jama*, 283(15), 2008–2012.

Tromski-Klingshirn, D. M., & Davis, T. E. (2007). Supervisees' perceptions of their clinical supervision: A study of the dual role of clinical and administrative supervisor. *Counselor Education and Supervision*, 46(4), 294–304.

Watkins, C. E. (2013). The beginnings of psychoanalytic supervision: The crucial role of Max Eitingon. *American Journal of Psychoanalysis*, 73(3), 254–270.

Watkins, C. E., Jr. (2018). The generic model of psychotherapy supervision: An analogized research-informing meta-theory. *Journal of Psychotherapy Integration*, 28(4), 521–536.

West, W., & Clark, V. (2004). Learnings from a qualitative study into counselling supervision: Listening to supervisor and supervisee. *Counselling and Psychotherapy Research*, 4(2), 20–26.

Wheeler, S., & Richards, K. (2007). The impact of clinical supervision on counsellors and therapists, their practice and their clients: A systematic review of the literature. *Counselling and Psychotherapy Research*, 7(1), 54–65.

Wilson, H. M., Davies, J. S., & Weatherhead, S. (2016). Trainee therapists' experiences of supervision during training: A meta-synthesis. *Clinical Psychology & Psychotherapy*, 23(4), 340–351.

Chapter 2

Effective supervision during the Covid-19 pandemic

The transition to remote learning

Liat Shklarski and Allison Abrams

Introduction

When we first started writing this book, we did not think to include a chapter about remote supervision. While it can be a common thing, specifically when it is done with supervisors and supervisees around the world, it did not seem to be relevant enough to warrant its own chapter. However, during the writing process, the Covid-19 pandemic completely changed the world's reality and our perception of remote learning, treatment, and socialization. The pandemic took away our sense of freedom. We no longer had the privilege of meeting our patients, our supervisors, or our supervisees in person. Almost overnight, we were required to shift our practices from face-to-face to video or phone sessions. Not only were we forced to change the frame and reconsider our work with patients, but we would also have to do the same with our supervisors.

What at first looked like a few weeks of practicing remotely soon turned into months. This raised many questions. Should I bring my comfortable office chair home or give up my office completely? Would there be any noticeable shift when moving from face-to-face to the computer? Would it change the dynamic between the supervisor and supervisee or affect the supervisee's educational experience?

Meeting face-to-face with either our patients or our supervisors did not seem likely to happen any time in the immediate future. Without much time to prepare ourselves—physically or psychologically—we had to swiftly find ways to adapt our clinical practices and our supervision with as little interruption as possible. Life as we knew it was disrupted enough, so it was crucial that we find ways to maintain as much stability in our professional lives as possible, particularly in our supervision.

As the format of supervision had changed, new adaptations were required, from finding a quiet spot that looked "professional" to figuring out the best platform on which to connect, working through technical issues (volume, screen, etc.), and note-taking. Shortly after the shelter-in-place order went into effect, we expressed to Barbara Stimmel our anxieties around helping our patients cope with this new reality. Many of these anxieties were the same as the ones our patients were struggling with, and this was something that none of us had ever experienced. We wondered how we could help if even we (the therapists) did not have the answers. We were just as lost as they were. There was an obvious parallel process taking place between us (the supervisees) and Barbara (the supervisor). Like our patients, we hoped she would offer reassurance and answers to so many of the questions we had. How will these circumstances change the therapeutic process? How do we reconceptualize therapy? This has never happened before—are we equipped to handle it? Will the work be as effective? Finally, how do we help our clients cope when we are still struggling to reconcile ourselves to this new reality?

When we brought these questions to our supervision sessions, Barbara insisted that this event was "no different" than any other traumatic event that a patient may have gone through, and that just because this specific event had never occurred before in our lifetimes it did not mean we were not equipped to help patients cope. Although certain adjustments needed to be made (transferring therapy to phone/video, being in each other's homes, etc.), the core of the work would not change. Rather than focus on the limitations, Barbara emphasized the fact that, yes, the frame, or the setting, had changed, but the work and the process, etc., had not. She said:

> The pandemic is a terrible reality. But the pandemic [per se] is not the issue. Talk to them [the patients] as if they are going through any other major life pressure—divorce, moving, etc. Each situation is unique, but your role and your responsiveness stay the same. Your attitude and approach remain the same. They have been through other traumas. This is no different. You as a therapist have the skills to help them cope with this trauma as you have helped patients deal with other traumas in their lives.

While acknowledging the very real reality of the situation and validating that, yes, none of us had ever gone through a global pandemic before, we should not have been thinking of the work any differently. Though technology has its challenges, conceptually, it does not change the essence of the work itself. Further, although the frame had changed, the therapeutic boundaries remained. But what if, for example, a patient's child or spouse came into the room during a therapy session? We wondered whether such things were going to be unavoidable under these unprecedented circumstances. Barbara insisted:

> You should still look at this clinically. If a patient showed up to your office with their child, you would not just ignore that. You would think about and talk to them about what it means. The patient could have made arrangements to have the session privately. She could have gone to her bedroom, rather than out in the living room. If the spouse was home, was it really impossible for them to have privacy for 45 minutes? Was this a resistance to the therapy? Was it resistance to asking their spouse for help—perhaps a

theme throughout their marriage? Do not think of the therapy any differently. You must still maintain the boundaries, with flexibility when necessary, but essentially the frame remains the same. Think about what it would mean if a patient showed up to a session in their pajamas, or even in bed. You are in their bed with them! What does that mean? If a patient showed up to your office wearing pajamas, you would analyze that.

Rationale for the current study

Barbara's opinion that we should not be thinking of the work any differently encouraged us to learn more about effective remote supervision during the pandemic. We reviewed the empirical literature about remote supervision and its effect on the quality of education provided. However, not many studies have addressed the topic. Needless to say, none focused on remote learning during a pandemic. Some studies focused on how or if the supervisory working alliance is influenced by the use of distance supervision (Bernhard & Camins, 2020; Inman et al., 2018; Watkins, 2014). And while research on distance supervision has taken place, much of it has focused on professionals' attitudes toward distance supervision (Conn et al., 2009; Munchel, 2015), trainee self-efficacy, and satisfaction with distance supervision (Erichsen et al., 2014).

For the purposes of this chapter, we decided to conduct a mixed-methods study with supervisees in order to answer the following questions: (1) What is the impact of the Covid-19 pandemic on the supervisory relationship and the effectiveness of supervision? (2) Does the use of technology to facilitate effective clinical supervision affect clinical supervision and the supervisory alliance?

Method

We used a sequential explanatory mixed-methods design to collect and analyze the data (Figure 2.1). The rationale for this was, first, to integrate the two methods to support each other in explaining and elaborating on the results and, second, to potentially foster theory building around the topic of effective supervision in transition time (to remote supervision and during a pandemic).

Participants

Eighty-five participants completed the survey. We had to exclude 11 participants who did not meet the following inclusion criteria: (1) currently in supervision; and (2) were in supervision before the pandemic (n = 76). The dataset was also restricted to the various items that were used as dependent variables. As Allison (2002) noted, there must be casewise deletion of missing data for any items that are used as dependent variables prior to all statistical calculations. Allison

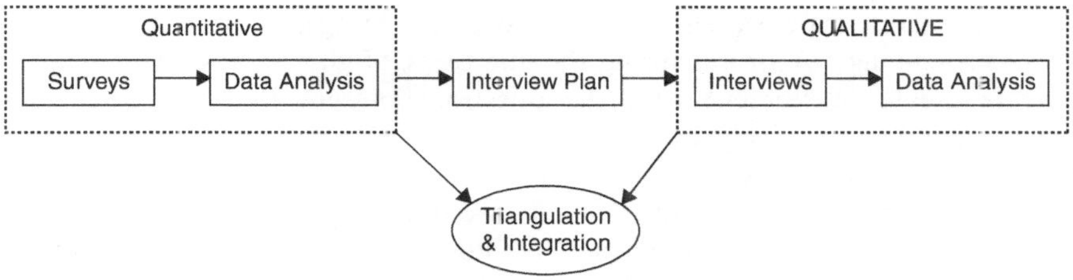

Figure 2.1 Sequential exploratory mixed-methods design
Source: Wu (2012).

further noted that this deletion is done because any imputation strategy for missing data on a dependent variable will cause inaccurate variance estimates of said dependent variable during an inferential statistical analysis procedure. The above procedures reduced the dataset from the original 85 cases to 76 cases, which represents a 1.06 percent attrition of cases.

The majority of participants were women holding a social work degree who ranged in age from 20 to 50 years (M = 36.6, SD = 1.073). They had seen clients and been supervised in the following settings: (1) private practice (51.2 percent); (2) not-for-profit agencies (28.8 percent); and (3) hospitals (20 percent). Participants had been in individual supervision with their supervisor for an average of 20 months (SD = 2.009).

Procedure

Following ethical approval from the Human Research and Ethics Committee of Long Island University (IRB Protocol #20/05–097), we recruited mental health professionals through dedicated professional listservs such as the New York State Society for Clinical Social Work, the Contemporary Freudian Society, and the International Network of Orthodox Mental Health Professionals. We sent a recruitment email that included a link to the survey. All participants signed an electronic informed consent form, which included a statement of ethics approval for the study as well as the goals of the research.

For the qualitative phase of the study, we used purposeful sampling (Suri, 2011). Specifically, we targeted individuals who had similar experiences before and during the pandemic and those who had negative experiences. We then contacted them to schedule a phone interview. Participants who took part in the semi-structured phone interview verbally consented to participate and to be recorded.

Measures/instrument

For the quantitative phase of the study, an anonymous, online survey asking 37 questions was developed to address the research questions. In the survey, we used Likert scale statements (e.g., strongly disagree, disagree, neutral, agree, strongly agree) for answering the questions. Higher scores on each scale indicate greater agreement with the questions present in each scale. The survey included positively and negatively worded questions which, during analysis, were reversed to increase consistency.

For the quantitative phase of the study, we developed an interview guide of 15 questions which was based on the literature review from Chapter 1. Cronbach's alpha was calculated to provide a measure of the internal consistency of a scale as a function of its reliability. The Cronbach's alpha was 0.725, which is an acceptable level of reliability.

Quantitative measures

Demographics

Demographic questions looked at the respondents' highest degree, sex, employment setting, and postgraduate training (see Table 2.1). Participants were also asked to describe the types of settings in which they had seen clients, the duration of individual supervision, the method used to meet with their supervisors before and during the pandemic, and the frequency of these supervision meetings. Finally, participants were asked to give their email address so that we could contact them to schedule the interview.

Effective supervision (dependent variable)

Effective supervision was measured by a set of eight questions to assess the working alliance between the participants and their supervisors. For example: "My supervisor has been able to support me in my work with clients during the pandemic," or "My working alliance with my supervisor did not change because of the pandemic."

Remote supervision (independent variable)

Participants were asked to report the platform they were using to meet with their supervisor. Seven additional questions assessed differences in remote versus in-person supervision. For example: "There is no difference between face-to-face and remote supervision," or "Supervision is less effective when done remotely."

Supervision during the pandemic (independent variable)

Participants were asked seven questions about their supervision experience during the pandemic. We emphasized changes that may have occurred in the supervisory relationship before and during the pandemic. For example: "My

Table 2.1 Quantitative participants: demographic characteristics, means, and standard deviation

Characteristic	*Number Quan*	*Mean Quan*	*SD*
Gender			
Female	62	81.6%	
Male	12	16%	
Non-binary	2	2.4%	
Age	76	36.6 years	1.073
20 to 29	18	23.7%	
30 to 39	25	32.9%	
40 to 49	22	28.9%	
50 to 59	8	10.5%	
60 and above	3	3.9%	
Highest level of education			
BA/BS	4	5.3%	
Master's degree	64	84.2%	
PhD/PsychD	8	10.5%	
Average time in supervision	76	1.95 years	2.009
Currently in postgraduate training	22	28.9%	
Discipline			
Social work	54	71.1%	
Other than social work	22	28.9%	

supervisor behaves the same during the pandemic," or "My relationship with my supervisor has changed since the pandemic began."

Qualitative measure

We developed the interview guide based on a literature review. The preliminary protocol was first piloted on two non-participant volunteers who met the participation criteria, and then altered based on the feedback. The protocol opened by giving participants a definition of effective supervision that was followed by questions related to their experiences in supervision before and during the pandemic. The next set of questions asked participants to describe changes in their relationships with their supervisors due to the transition to remote supervision. The interview closed by asking participants what they would recommend a young clinician look for when seeking a supervisor.

Data analysis

Procedures for analyzing quantitative data

We used the Statistical Package for the Social Sciences program to analyze the quantitative data. First, we conducted reverse coding to make sure that all numerical scoring scales were in the same direction. We descriptively analyzed the data in order to demonstrate the shape, central tendency, and variability within the dataset. Percentages and frequencies were calculated for all categorical variables and means, and standard deviations were calculated for all continuous variables. Next, we conducted a correlation analysis between the dependent variable and the independent variables. In particular, we conducted a bivariate Pearson correlation to measure the following associations and correlations among pairs of variables and between sets of variables. The bivariate Pearson correlation indicates whether a statistically significant linear relationship exists between continuous variables that measured the independent and dependent variables and the direction of a linear relationship (increasing or decreasing). We also conducted independent samples t-tests and used one-way analysis of variance to assess the difference between the means of two (or more) independent groups. Lastly, we conducted multiple linear regression between the dependent variable and the independent variables. The omnibus F-test was statistically significant ($F = 2.700$; $df = 13, 62$; $p < 0.01$). Among the 13 independent predictor variables, only three emerged as statistically significant predictors of the first dependent variable.

Procedures for analyzing the qualitative data

Thematic analysis was undertaken (Braun & Clarke, 2012). In this process, we transcribed the recorded interviews and read them to identify concepts. After repeating these steps across all transcripts, emerging codes and categories were compared between two reviewers (the researchers), connected as appropriate, and organized into key concepts. Later, we used a member check-in method to check the trustworthiness of the interpreted data (Birt et al., 2016).

Results

Remote supervision

In this study, 88.2 percent of the participants met their supervisors in person before the pandemic and then switched to remote supervision that was either on the phone (n = 37, 48 percent) or used a combined method (n = 39, 51.3 percent). The preference in terms of video platform was either FaceTime or Zoom. Participants in our study reported an overall positive relationship with their supervisor: 82 percent of participants rated their relationship as good to very good, and 76.4 percent either agreed or strongly agreed with the statement "I like my supervisor's personality."

We noticed that there was a difference in perceived effective supervision between participants who worked in private practice settings as opposed to nonprofit settings. A positive association was found between the quality of supervision among participants in private practice ($r = 0.33$, $p < 0.0005$), and there was a negative correlation between the two among participants who worked in nonprofit settings ($r = 0.68$, $p < 0.0005$).

Our findings suggest that remote supervision can be as effective as face-to-face modes. A positive association was found between the quality of supervision using remote tools and participants' agreement with there being "no change" in their working alliance when they met with their supervision in person ($r = -0.84$, $p < 0.0005$). However, the multiple regression analysis shows that participants favored meeting in person ($B = 0.419$, $p < 0.001$). Between the different platforms used to conduct remote supervision, using FaceTime leads to lower scores of effective supervision ($B = -0.371$, $p < 0.05$). Lastly, a negative unstandardized coefficient relates to the age of the participant; younger participants perceived remote supervision as less effective ($B = -0.148$, $p < 0.05$).

There was a negative association between remote supervision and its effectiveness ($r = -0.47$, $p < 0.0005$). Participants did not report an association between remote supervision (such as phone, video, or combined) and the effectiveness of supervision. While there was no statistically significant association between the platform used (phone, video, or combined), the results show that participants who used the combined method (video and phone) rated the supervision as less effective.

In order to assess the relationship between effective supervision and the working alliance, we conducted a Pearson's correlation (see Table 2.2). There was a moderate positive correlation between participants who reported that their supervisor behaved the same before and during the pandemic and how they rated their relationship with their supervisor ($r = 0.49$, $p < 0.0005$). Participants were asked to rate the quality of their relationship with their supervisors. Consistency in their supervisors' behavior (before and during the pandemic) accounts for 40 percent of the variation in participants' ratings of the quality of their supervision ($r = 0.60$, $p < 0.0005$).

As the quantitative data show, participants did not always feel that there was a significant difference between in-person and remote supervision. The qualitative data provide insight into the potential disruptions and changes that occur in the transition to remote supervision. We divided the data into two categories: (1) the structure and frame of remote supervision; and (2) technological proficiency of the supervisor.

The structure and frame of remote supervision

Following the quantitative results, the findings show that remote supervision can be effective. In particular, participants stated that in order to increase its effectiveness, the structure of the meetings should be accommodated to suit the online platform. For example, in some cases, participants and their supervisors had a prior conversation in regard to the platform to be used, the physical space, and confidentiality. Participant AJ explained: "Supervision virtually doesn't have to be less effective overall—in fact, I think it's just as effective, but the structure and frame needs to be thought about in terms of the differences to in-person supervision."

What seems to be natural engagement in the office changes in remote meetings. As a result, the frame should be accommodated according to the new format. On the other hand, some participants expressed concerns about the new structure of remote supervision. Specifically, that remote supervision was not as formal as in-person meetings. Participant HG explained: "There are elements that are missing virtually that I felt were present in person—like the formality or the amount of preparation I brought to the sessions." Another profound example of the need to adjust the frame was shared by a music therapist who described the unique struggle of transitioning music therapy from in-person to remote: "Creative arts-based supervision has become how to navigate the different ways we can do music therapy. Not to replicate it necessarily, but how to make use of what we have, with the limited options we have." He continued, "It has been a learning process of 'rolling with the punches' by doing less arts-based supervision, which is more challenging." This may relate to the external and internal distractions that occur before and during meetings with supervisors. Participant CM answered the question "How is it for you to do remote supervision?" by explaining:

> I hate it. I mean, I've been doing it throughout but it's been hard for me to stay focused in the beginning, not as much, but as time goes on more and more difficult. I find my mind wandering. I find if it's on a phone, sometimes I hear the beeps of my WhatsApp.

In this case, while the frame was discussed in advance, many distractions still came up along the way that affected the quality of the supervision. Forms of distractions in this case related to the supervisee, but in another case, participant AJ described their supervisor as the one who appeared to be distracted: "The real difference is that she [the supervisor] is not as focused. I find like I've seen her texting other people during my supervision and I didn't say anything."

It seems as if internal and external distractions will always be present. Nevertheless, both supervisors and supervisees should make a conscious effort to create a setup that is comfortable for each of them, as if they were meeting in the office. Participant JM brings up some of her personal versus professional conflicts in regard to the platform she is using with her supervisor—specifically, her challenges with supervision via FaceTime, which she had always associated with personal relationships: "Pre-pandemic, I primarily used FaceTime with close family members and loved ones, in bed, saying goodnight to a partner away on a trip, with a glass of wine."

FaceTime is no longer used only for personal connections but for work purposes as well, which requires making certain internal adjustments. To add to that, some participants described the differences in meeting with their supervisor over the phone as opposed to on a video chat. Some participants found the video platform to be more effective than the phone. Participant GH explained: "I prefer to meet her [supervisor] either by FaceTime or Zoom, just because I really like to see facial expressions. As a clinician, you get much more information from people when you see them face-to-face."

Technological proficiency of the supervisor

While we did not ask a question about their perceptions of their supervisors' proficiency with technology and its effect on the quality of supervision, the participants reported feeling frustrated when their supervisors did not know how to use technology. They reported that, as a result, the supervisor was more distracted, troubleshooting took more time, and the supervision was shorter. As participant XM explained:

> My supervisor had never used video conferencing before, so it was a learning process for him. He had a lot of difficulty with it at first, which ended up cutting into much of the supervision session time. Needless to say, this affected the effectiveness of supervision and contributed to the already existing stress of the situation.

Both supervisors and supervisees, to some degree, need technological support. The transition to remote supervision and treatment was abrupt due to the pandemic, and, as a result, there was no time to prepare or to "practice" using the new platforms. Some participants shared that they did not encounter any technical issues, and that their supervisors were proficient enough to the point that they could support them. Participant RC reported several advantages to having a technologically proficient supervisor. When she complained to her supervisor about her challenges with remote therapy, her supervisor helped her make necessary adjustments to accommodate the remote setting, both explicitly and implicitly:

> She tried to have her own home office set up in a professional way. For example, she helped me to be more aware of moving the camera further out so that I could see part of her body and not just her face close up.

RC's supervisor helped her refine other aspects as well, such as shifting her gaze—"as we do in person. We are not always staring right at them, we look away at times"—and other forms of virtual etiquette: "She modeled that in an implicit way, which registered."

These examples highlight how important it is to be aware of the elements of technology that influence the effectiveness of the supervisory meeting—

Table 2.2 Statistically significant correlations: remote supervision

Dependent variables	*Independent variables*	*Sig.*
Rate the quality of your supervision	Q19. Supervision is less effective when supervision is done remotely.	−475**
Rate the quality of your supervision	Q23. There is no difference between face-to-face and remote supervision.	336**
Rate the quality of your supervision	Q29. Supervision became less formal because of remote learning (as opposed to in-person meetings).	−464**
Rate your relationship with your supervisor		−301**
Rate the quality of your supervision	Q30. Supervision became less effective because of remote learning (as opposed to in-person meetings).	−723**
Rate your relationship with your supervisor		−0.392**

Note: ** Correlation is significant at the 0.01 level (2-tailed).

elements that we did not have to think about when we were sitting in the office together.

Supervision during the pandemic

Overall, the supervisory relationship was not significantly affected by the pandemic, and 76.6 percent of the participants kept meeting with their supervisors in the same capacity that they used to meet prior to the pandemic. As a matter of fact, 60 percent of the participants reported that they urgently needed to meet with their supervisor during the pandemic (M = 2.65, SD = 0.684), and 80 percent of the participants reported that their supervisors had been able to support them in their work with clients during the pandemic (M = 4.19, SD = 1.03).

Effective supervision during the pandemic was correlated with a positive supervisory relationship (see Table 2.3). For example, there was a positive correlation between the stability of the working alliance prior to the pandemic and the quality of supervision during the pandemic ($r = 50$, $p < 0.0005$): 63 percent of participants disagreed with the statement "My relationship with my supervisor has changed since the pandemic began," and 20 percent were neutral about this statement (M = 2.2, SD = 1.2); 75 percent of participants also relatively disagreed with the statement "Since the pandemic started, supervision has felt less effective" (M = 2.09, SD = 0.856).

Some 70 percent of participants reported that, overall, their supervisors were behaving the same during the pandemic. While 40 percent of participants reported that their supervisor was more laid back during the pandemic, there was a negative correlation between effective supervision and participants' rating of their supervisor as more laid back during the pandemic ($r = -0.30$, $p < 0.0005$). This

Table 2.3 Statistically significant correlations: pandemic

Dependent variables	*Independent variables*	*Sig.*
Rate the quality of your supervision	Q27. My professional and personal stress due to the pandemic has affected the quality of my supervision.	−0.386**
Rate the quality of your supervision	Q17. My supervisor is more laid back during the pandemic.	−0.304**
Rate your relationship with your supervisor		−231*
Rate the quality of your supervision	Q18. My supervisor is less consistent during the pandemic.	−0.367**
Rate your relationship with your supervisor		−303**
Rate the quality of your supervision	Q16. My supervisor behaves the same during the pandemic.	0.641**
Rate your relationship with your supervisor		0.492**
Rate the quality of your supervision	Q25. Since the pandemic started, supervision has felt less effective.	−401**
Rate your relationship with your supervisor		−390**
Rate the quality of your supervision	Q34. My supervisor has been able to support me in my work with clients during the pandemic.	0.735**
Rate your relationship with your supervisor		0.539**
Rate the quality of your supervision	Q32. My working alliance with my supervisor did not change because of the pandemic.	0.504**
Rate your relationship with your supervisor		−468**
Rate the quality of your supervision	Q20. My relationship with my supervisor has changed since the pandemic began.	−0.456**
Rate your relationship with your supervisor		−313**

Notes: ** Correlation is significant at the 0.01 level (2-tailed).

* Correlation is significant at the 0.05 level (2-tailed).

finding is supported by the negative association we found between participants' ratings of their supervisors as less consistent during the pandemic and the positive quality of their relationships with their supervisors ($r = -0.36$, $p < 0.0005$). In other words, participants who rated their relationships as positive reported that their supervisors were consistent during the pandemic.

The findings are consistent, and there is a positive correlation between supervisors' consistent behaviors during the pandemic and the supervisees' level of satisfaction with the supervisory relationship (r = 0.49, p <0.0005). Regardless of the pandemic and the transition to remote supervision, the relationship with the supervisor is a key component in the quality of supervision (r = 60, p <0.0005).

We asked participants about their own personal and professional stress and how it affected their supervision experiences. There was no single response that stood out from the others. Overall, participants tended to stay neutral to this statement (M = 2.74, SD = 1.323). Nevertheless, there was a negative correlation between positive supervisory relationships and high levels of professional and personal stress because of the pandemic. Those who rated their relationship with their supervisor as satisfactory reported that their supervisory relationship was less affected by their stress (r = −0.38, p <0.0005).

It seems that, overall, the supervisory relationship did not change; however, the qualitative data provide a more detailed explanation of the changes. We divided the qualitative data related to effective supervision during the pandemic into five categories: (1) the structure of the supervision meetings; (2) addressing the changes; (3) balancing the personal and the professional in the supervisory relationship; (4) the content of supervision; and (5) power dynamics.

Structure

Participants emphasized the change in structure because of the pandemic. Participant RS spoke about the importance of structure to ensuring effective supervision: "Having structure in general is helpful. Just knowing it's a consistent thing, as it generally was [pre-pandemic]." In fact, since the pandemic, she stated that she and her supervisor had been sticking to that same time and day even more than they usually had: "It is something that I know I have built into my schedule." Perhaps having the consistency and structure remain the same provides a sense of stability in an overwhelmingly unstable time, both personally and professionally.

For some, because of the pandemic, a lot of the structure was disturbed by other personal and professional obligations. Participant GH explained:

> Sometimes because of the last-minute schedule changes, it sounds like it's easier for my supervisor to just have a phone session instead of the video sessions. And that's been something that I think has diminished the quality of the supervision a little bit.

Due to the pandemic, supervisors' and supervisees' priorities changed. Suddenly, schools closed and everyone was at home together. Mental health professionals are considered first responders and are needed to work extra time. Inevitably, the structure changed, which impacted the effectiveness of the supervision. Participant LM added that the structure had to change because of other professional obligations as well as personal matters such as child care. She explained:

> We used to have our supervision sessions during the day. But now, because she's [supervisor] homeschooling her children and I had to start working additional hours because of Covid-19, we had to move our supervision sessions to later in the evenings which was sometimes problematic. People's schedules are different now.

The pandemic added an additional challenge to the structure, which is doing the work from our own homes. Very few participants reported conducting remote sessions from their offices or said that their supervisors were sitting in their offices. The majority of the participants and their supervisors worked from home, specifically because of the shelter-in-place orders that prevented people from leaving their homes. Participant OT explained:

> There are logistical challenges because I work from home, my kids are home, and she [supervisor] was sick with Covid so we could not connect. It is a lot harder to connect with her because she is out of the city. She has her personal stuff and I do not feel as supported at all. Sometimes we can't do FT so we do the phone but I do not connect as well. It does not feel the same.

The structure has changed because of many variables that are not in the control of the supervisee or the supervisor. It has been a time of adaptation for everyone, and this has affected the effectiveness of the supervision as a result.

Addressing the changes

Participants highlighted their need to process the effects of the pandemic on their personal and professional lives in supervision. They found supervision to be more effective when there was a discussion about the global problem. Participants were specifically asked about what would make supervision more effective during the pandemic. Participant AS explained: "Acknowledging the reality of the pandemic and the uncertainty." Similarly, participant VB stated: "Authenticity and genuine recognition of the situation."

Participants did not want their supervisors to take a "business as usual approach" when the pandemic occurred. There was an expectation that accommodations in the supervisory relationship would be made in response to this unique and painful situation. As participant AW explained:

> Like the clinical work, I think supervision has to reflect and acknowledge the changing circumstances, not attempt to recreate what we had before. I think that working with that has been the most successful part of my supervision and my work so far. I think that what has made my supervision effective is that my supervisor asks more about how I'm doing and helps me navigate how to respond to patients in their worries about me.

To this same point, participant RS stated:

> It seems crazy not to acknowledge the reality of the changes we are all living through, the chaos, and the uncertainty, but not to overprocess it to the detriment of talking about the details of cases and getting feedback on interventions.

Further, she said:

> People need to process a lot of the reality. We can't just stick our heads in the sand. We need to hold off on the hardcore interpreting because people just need to find their bearings. This is reflected in our supervision work as well. We're building this plane as we're flying it.

Aside from the need to address the global crisis, some participants reported that they needed to learn how to support themselves, their families, and their patients who presented with new, unfamiliar issues. Participant MJ explained that this pertained to: "The loss of life, the loss of feeling in control, feeling effective, and how to deal with people in the face of all that loss and be the one that can be the helper." In her opinion, her supervisor became more effective when he could adhere to the new reality and support her in finding ways to support her patients while she was facing personal challenges. This notion was supported by another participant who felt that the pandemic required her to develop new clinical skills. Participant FN thought that effective supervision during the pandemic should focus on generating new interventions to support patients: "It would be helpful if current supervision targeted the ongoing climate with specific interventions and theories to support clinicians in treating patients."

Balancing the personal and the professional in the supervisory relationship

The distinction between personal and professional material in supervision is a topic that is often discussed in the literature and research on supervision (Davys & Beddoe, 2010; Jordan & Shearer, 2019; Yegdich, 1999). During the pandemic, drawing this delicate line became an issue requiring closer attention and further discussion. At times, the boundaries of supervision became blurred and began to feel more like therapy. "It's striking a new balance between the personal and the professional," stated participant RS. "Supervision is not therapy, but it is also not 100 percent not therapy. There is more flexibility in the frame than there would be in therapy."

Participant FL added that, because of the pandemic, it is inevitable that personal experiences will be discussed during supervision:

> Just trying to hold some balance of the frame when really the frame has been so ridiculously stretched. I feel that there's almost a loosening of this frame and

> supervision as well. So much of my personal life is coming up more in supervision because of the realities of what's been going on with this pandemic and the losses that I've had and the losses that my patients have had.

Most participants appreciated when their supervisors acknowledged the current circumstances and the challenges they brought up on both personal and professional levels, as opposed to diving into the clinical material without addressing them in the larger context of a global pandemic. Participant MJ explained:

> Since the pandemic started, I have been emotionally and physically vulnerable, but also in terms of my work, just my own feeling if I am helpful or effective. Being able to speak about that in supervision is something that I've been addressing in new ways.

She continued, "I think the lines between supervision and therapy are always very tenuous and not so distinct, but more so now than ever, it's impossible to separate it in the way that maybe before I thought I could."

Effective supervision during the pandemic no longer solely focuses on clinical material but also on refining the balance between personal and professional content. Participant BH, who had been meeting with her supervisor in her supervisor's office prior to the pandemic, stated: "I couldn't shake the feeling of being a patient; sitting in the waiting room, waiting to be called in. As a new clinician, my associations [to the therapy office] have always been as a client." She remained attuned to some of the overlaps and how to navigate the relationship between supervisor and supervisee as separate from but also related to the therapeutic relationship:

> When we worked in her office, I was very aware of my position and was mindful of that power imbalance. It was my supervisor's office, her time, you get up and leave, and in that way, it sometimes felt not as comfortable.

Once the format changed, so too did the power dynamic within the relationship. "Since we have been working via FaceTime, it has felt much more like peer-to-peer communication ... there's something very intimate about FaceTime in terms of the glitchiness of it and having to navigate that and being in someone's home." She gave an example of when each of their pets came into view on the screen, a common occurrence in remote sessions: "We swapped pictures of our cats over text, which we wouldn't have done before [the pandemic]."

In many cases, participants reported that they spent more time at the beginning of the supervision sessions "checking in" on personal matters (related to Covid-19, adjustment, and difficulties around the pandemic). Participant AA described feeling closer and more connected to her supervisor in part because of the informality: "We are going through the same thing. It is a bonding experience where we are holding these very expansive emotions." She found the informality to be beneficial, and that it increased the effectiveness of the supervision because "the change brought about more conversations about where we were both at, managing clients during the pandemic. It became a more vulnerable space." Further, she described finding a "balance between dealing with the external and internal reality of clients' cases and talking more about our family's health, what it's like, our own anxiety, and digesting and metabolizing all the unknowns we are navigating."

Content of supervision

In Chapter 1, we discussed the concept of supervision as a safe space. In some cases, the global crisis has made the supervisory relationship stronger mainly because of the collective experience. Participant HL explained that her supervisor shows more empathy toward the situation:

> I feel that she is really sympathetic to my situation as a learner and makes significant efforts to support me in this process so that I am still able to embrace the challenges and learning opportunities that present themselves. I feel like the content of our sessions together involves anxieties about remote services and some difficulties with conducting telehealth for residents of shelters.

These may not have been relevant topics of conversation before the pandemic, but they have definitely become the main topics during this time.

Power dynamics

Several participants described the supervisory relationship as feeling less hierarchical, which one hospital social work intern experienced as both a positive and a negative. She enjoyed not having the hierarchical dynamic, stating: "It was a confidence booster to feel more like colleagues." On the other hand, she also felt she missed the structure of the hierarchy:

> It was less helpful because it was a very overwhelming period. Survival is first. I was raised by immigrant parents. An old-school hierarchy exists, the student has their place, lower than the supervisor. I am there to learn. I'm lower on the totem pole.

Similarly, participant RC also noticed a shift in the hierarchy between her and her supervisor, whom she began to see as more of a human being, which was valuable to her.

> I have had other supervisors in the past who I felt I had to impress and appear to be doing a good job, that's part of the dynamic. But transitioning to remote

> dismantled that a little bit. You can see more of their true selves …. It is less hierarchical, because two people are coming together on this platform, and we are all dealing with these things in the world.

For her, having less of a hierarchy has had a more positive effect: "I like to feel that supervisors are fallible." Similarly, participant BR, who had a long-standing relationship with her supervisor, perceived the shift in power dynamics as "extremely beneficial" during this time, as she has felt more comfortable being open and expressing her feelings and talking about challenges related to the pandemic.

Discussion

The current study supports previous findings presenting some of the challenges likely to come up when conducting remote supervision, including distractions in the physical setting, confidentiality and ethical issues, technological problems, and others (Bender & Dykeman, 2016; Bernhard & Camins, 2020; Bruce et al., 2018; Fishkin et al., 2011; Kanz, 2001; Martin, 2018; Martin et al., 2017). Our participants agreed that conducting supervision from behind a computer screen presents its own challenges. As it is with therapy, it can never replace two people being in the room together.

Despite its limitations, the evidence suggests that remote learning can be as effective as (and sometimes more effective than) face-to-face modes (Bender & Dykeman, 2016; Oliaro & Trotter, 2010, as cited in Rushton et al., 2017). This has been shown in this study as well. In most cases, the transition to remote supervision did not affect the supervisory relationship or its effectiveness. Participants in our study reported that their relationships with their supervisors did not change when they used the phone versus a video platform. However, using a combination of phone and video had a slight impact on supervision's effectiveness. This finding highlights the need for consistency and a solid structure in order to better improve the communication between supervisors and supervisees and master one form of technology.

Participants reported that the majority of issues with remote supervision related to external distractions, such as hearing or seeing a text message or incoming email notifications while in supervision, and the connection also froze at times, which made it more difficult. It was more challenging to build an authentic relationship with supervisors because there was some disconnect caused by video chats or phone calls, and at times this resulted in an inability to visualize body language and other visual cues. Our participants reported that a strong rapport with their supervisors was key to effective supervision.

While participants did not favor the remote method (as opposed to in-person), they perceived supervision to be a valuable tool for their professional development, and, as a result, they chose to maintain it in its remote format. The supervision remained meaningful, challenging, helpful, and deep.

The second component of this study investigated effective supervision during the pandemic. Our findings show that while the effectiveness of supervision was not severely compromised, there were many elements that required additional awareness and adaptations. Both in the quantitative and qualitative inquiries, participants reported some change in the structure of supervision. Aside from the inevitable change to remote supervision and the replacement of the office environment with home, the supervisory hour had significantly changed because of the supervisor and supervisee. Participants reported a longer "check-in" taking place at the beginning of the meeting with their supervisor. It was no longer a generic "how are you?" but an inquiry into how each was coping with an unbearable situation in which they were both trying to keep their heads above water during a very challenging time.

Participants still found the supervision meetings to be effective, but they reported that their supervisors were more laid back and slightly less formal. In some cases, the participants reported that they had forgotten to log in to the sessions at times, were less organized than normal, and less prepared. The personal aspect of the working relationship between the supervisor and the supervisee had grown stronger because of the unique circumstances.

Participants highlighted that the inevitable changes in their personal lives (and their supervisors' lives) significantly changed the structure of their supervision. Suddenly, there were other things that each party needed to take care of: children, homeschooling, Covid-19 sickness, struggling with the loss of loved ones, the shelter-in-place order, going to the grocery store, taking care of elderly parents, and taking care of patients and students. Also, on a professional level, there were elevated anxieties about remote services and some difficulties with conducting telehealth. These may not have been relevant topics of conversation before the pandemic, but they have definitely become topics of urgency.

As a result, participants have felt less focused, less sharp, and at times they have not been able to remember as much because of pandemic-related sleep dysregulation, stress, and anxiety. Although at times participants have felt as though personal stressors may distract from the focus of the supervision, these conversations have led to discussions relevant to the pandemic in connection to their clinical work.

The pandemic created a condition in which everything had to be done remotely. The combination of providing remote therapy with additional computer time has been challenging. Participants appreciate that their supervisors have been able to accommodate the frame, recognize the difficulties, and work around them. It was almost impossible to jump right into the clinical material without first addressing and processing some of the personal issues related to the pandemic.

Implications for practice and future research

We are writing this chapter during what looks like the first wave of Covid-19 without really knowing if there will be a second wave, if we will return to the office, or for how long we will be conducting supervisory meetings remotely. While one part of us is missing our offices, Barbara's office, the commute, our "regular" lives, another is getting used to the new reality and finding the good in it. This uncertainty prompts us to reflect on the "new normal" and recommend new practices and preparation for remote supervision. Our participants would benefit from more concrete guidelines on how to conduct remote supervision, as would we. Some of these guidelines are being formed (Hames et al., 2020), but there is a need to study the topic so we can provide empirical evidence for effective remote supervision. For example, who calls who? On what platform? How can we mute notifications? Where should we station the computer? How can we cope with background noise? All of that has been learned on the spot. However, it is not too late to have conversations about it and generate additional research on how to enhance effective supervision both during and after the Covid-19 pandemic of 2020.

Limitations of the current study

Our analysis did not include variations between the different health professions and work settings, and it would be interesting to know whether the effectiveness of supervision varies between mental health professionals who work in private practice, hospitals, clinics, etc. As a matter of fact, the independent t-test to examine an association between effective supervision and work setting did show that participants working in nonprofit settings found remote supervision to be less effective than those in private practice. Therefore, a further examination of effective remote supervision in nonprofit agencies is necessary.

We assessed effective supervision during the pandemic with the goal of observing any possible effects of the pandemic on supervision, but our study is limited because it did not gather information about effective supervision prior to the pandemic. We recommend assessing the influence of the pandemic on effective supervision by conducting a pre–post design (during the pandemic and after).

While we would have liked to have spent more time learning about the participants' adjustments in a more specific way by going back to the very first few sessions after shelter-in-place orders were issued, instead, we asked them about their overall experiences. A more detailed inquiry would be beneficial to understand the transitions and the mechanisms in place that helped to retain the effectiveness of the supervisory relationship. Moreover, our sample was a convenience sample—the majority of the participants were located in the tri-state area of New York, and most were social workers in private practice. As a result, our sample is lacking the randomization and accuracy that is so important when conducting research. It is also important in the context of understanding the relationship between effective supervision and the pandemic, mainly because some states have been affected more than others; it would be interesting to learn about the experiences of participants from other states that were not as affected by Covid-19 as New York.

Lastly, since the majority of our participants were social workers, we wonder how remote supervision and the pandemic have affected the supervisory relationships of clinicians from other disciplines, specifically, psychologists, psychiatrists, and psychoanalysts. The anecdotal evidence shows that clinicians' experiences have been similar across disciplines. Nevertheless, there is room to replicate this study with a heterogeneous population.

Conclusions

With advances in technology making it easier than ever to connect, opportunities to work remotely in therapy as well as in supervision are abundant. Platforms such as email and video conferencing permit practitioners to "bridge distances" (Goodyear & Rousmaniere, 2019) in both the literal and figurative sense. Whether for geographical reasons or as an adaptation to disruptions in our lives—as in the case of the Covid-19 pandemic—technology proves to be the ultimate solution to bridging these gaps and sustaining the effective clinical supervision of mental health professionals across disciplines and theoretical schools.

In contrast to Barbara's insistence that the pandemic is no different from any other trauma that we help our clients through, many of the participants reported that what stuck with them was in fact the idea we are all experiencing the same trauma simultaneously. This pertains to our work with clients as well as with our supervisors. This brings us to the conclusion of this chapter, which is that since the pandemic is such a unique situation, there is a need for additional research on and the development of new practices to address our new lives with Covid-19.

After completing the surveys and at the end of the interviews, the participants thanked us for conducting such an important study. At first, it felt like they were merely extending to us the usual courtesy; but when we analyzed the data, we became aware of the significant amount of suffering that was being discussed for perhaps the first time in our semi-structured interviews. We even received an email from one participant who shared that the interview had made her reflect on the structure of her supervision and led her to successfully advocate that her clinic change the work setting from phone to video, which she would not have thought to do prior to participating in our study.

In response to stressors, our bodies and minds enter fight or flight mode, and our responses to this pandemic have demonstrated this natural reaction. As clinicians and supervisees, we did not have the luxury of time to process what was happening during the initial outbreak of Covid-19, so we just kept going in order to survive. Our study invited supervisees to pause, think, reflect, mourn, and feel frustrated and thankful for their ability to maintain successful working relationships with their supervisors during an unfamiliar and painful collective experience that will be a significant part of the history books!

References

Allison, P. D. (2002). *Quantitative applications in the social sciences: Missing data*. SAGE Publications. doi:10.4135/9781412985079.

Bender, S., & Dykeman, C. (2016). Supervisees' perceptions of effective supervision: A comparison of fully synchronous cybersupervision to traditional methods. *Journal of Technology in Human Services*, 34(4), 326–337.

Bernhard, P. A., & Camins, J. S. (2020). Supervision from afar: Trainees' perspectives on telesupervision. *Counselling Psychology Quarterly*. doi:doi:10.1080/09515070.2020.1770697.

Birt, L., Scott, S., Cavers, D., Campbell, C., & Walter, F. (2016). Member checking: A tool to enhance trustworthiness or merely a nod to validation? *Qualitative Health Research*, 26(13), 1802–1811. doi:10.1177/1049732316654870.

Braun, V., & Clarke, V. (2012). Thematic analysis. In H. Cooper, P. M. Camic, D. L. Long, A. T. Panter, D. Rindskopf, & K. J. Sher (Eds.), APA handbooks in psychology. *APA handbook of research methods in psychology, Vol. 2. Research designs: Quantitative, qualitative, neuropsychological, and biological* (pp. 57–71). American Psychological Association. doi:10.1037/13620-004.

Bruce, T., Byrne, F., & Kemp, L. (2018). Using Skype to support remote clinical supervision for health professionals delivering a sustained maternal early childhood programme: A phenomenographical study. *Contemporary Nurse*, 54(1), 4–12.

Conn, S. R., Roberts, R. L., & Powell, B. M. (2009). Attitudes and satisfaction with a hybrid model of counseling supervision. *Journal of Educational Technology & Society*, 12(2), 298–306.

Davys, A., & Beddoe, L. (2010). *Best practice in professional supervision: A guide for the helping professions*. Jessica Kingsley.

Erichsen, E. A., Bolliger, D. U., & Halupa, C. (2014). Student satisfaction with graduate supervision in doctoral programs primarily delivered in distance education settings. *Studies in Higher Education*, 39(2), 321–338.

Fishkin, R., Fishkin, L., Leli, U., Katz, B., & Snyder, E. (2011). Psychodynamic treatment, training, and supervision using internet-based technologies. *Journal of the American Academy of Psychoanalysis and Dynamic Psychiatry*, 39(1), 155–168.

Goodyear, R. K., & Rousmaniere, T. (2019). Introduction: Computer and internet-based technologies for psychotherapy, supervision, and supervision-of-supervision. *Journal of Clinical Psychology*, 75 (2), 243–246.

Hames, J. L., Bell, D. J., Perez-Lima, L. M., Holm-Denoma, J. M., Rooney, T., Charles, N. E., … & Simmons, K. T. (2020). Navigating uncharted waters: Considerations for training clinics in the rapid transition to telepsychology and telesupervision during COVID-19. *Journal of Psychotherapy Integration*, 30(2), 348–365.

Inman, A. G., Soheilian, S. A., & Luu, L. P. (2018). Telesupervision: Building bridges in a digital era. *Journal of Clinical Psychology*, 75, 292–301.

Jordan, S. E., & Shearer, E. M. (2019). An exploration of supervision delivered via clinical video telehealth (CVT). *Training and Education in Professional Psychology*, 13(4), 323–330.

Kanz, J. E. (2001). Clinical-supervision.com: Issues in the provision of online supervision. *Professional Psychology: Research and Practice*, 32(4), 415–420. doi:10.1037/0735-7028.32.4.415.

Martin, P. (2018). Clinical supervision in the bush: Is it any different? *International Journal of Integrated Care (IJIC)*, 18, 2–12.

Martin, P., Kumar, S., & Lizarondo, L. (2017). Effective use of technology in clinical supervision. *Internet Interventions*, 8, 35–39.

Munchel, F. (2015) *Exploratory Study of Counseling Professionals' Attitudes toward Distance Clinical Supervision* [Unpublished doctoral dissertation]. University of South Florida. http://scholarcommons.usf.edu/etd/5997.

Rushton, J., Hutchings, J., Shepherd, K., & Douglas, J. (2017). Zooming in: Social work supervisors using online supervision. *Aotearoa New Zealand Social Work*, 29 (3), 126–130.

Suri, H. (2011). Purposeful sampling in qualitative research synthesis. *Qualitative Research Journal*, 11(2), 63–75.

Watkins, C. E. (2014). The supervisory alliance as quintessential integrative variable. *Journal of Contemporary Psychotherapy*, 44(3), 151–161.

Wu, P. F. (2012). A mixed methods approach to technology acceptance research. *Journal of the Association for Information Systems*, 13(3), 172–187.

Yegdich, T. (1999). Lost in the crucible of supportive clinical supervision: Supervision is not therapy. *Journal of Advanced Nursing*, 29(5), 1265–1275.

Chapter 3

Social justice and cultural competence in clinical supervision

Liat Shklarski and Allison Abrams

Introduction

In the last several decades, just as the field of mental health counseling has expanded and evolved around the globe, so too has the field of clinical supervision. Specifically, this expansion has occurred across countries, cultures, theoretical approaches, and venues, resulting in the production of empirical and theoretical literature focusing on cultural differences between the supervisor and the supervisee as an important component affecting the quality of the supervisory relationship (Akkurt et al., 2018; Estrada, 2018; Hird et al., 2001). No longer a process confined to a room in which a supervisor and supervisee meet face-to-face, given globalization and advances in technology, supervision today can take place between clinicians living on opposite sides of the world.

Since this book's contributors come from diverse cultures and different countries, we knew that we wanted to include a chapter on cultural competence in supervision. When we initially invited the contributors to participate in the book, our conversations with them about their experiences in supervision were fascinating. It became clear that in addition to the cultural competence variable was an important mediating variable in the form of the setting in which the supervision took place (particularly in the cases of three analysts who started their work with Barbara Stimmel in person and transitioned to remote). The anecdotal evidence indicated that the cultural competence variable could be mediated by the setting and actually influenced the effectiveness of supervision.

We believe that in order to start a conversation about culturally competent supervision, we should first address an equally significant partner: social justice. To achieve true cultural competence in supervision, it is essential that supervisors not only have an understanding of cultural differences but that they are also educated on and sensitive to societal inequalities (Fickling et al., 2019). This chapter will first address the topic of social justice and its implications for effective supervision. Next, we will elaborate on cultural competence in cross-cultural supervision. We will then explore cross-cultural supervision between Western supervisors and supervisees from Asia, reflecting the examples of cases included in this book. Finally, we will discuss recommendations for the further advancement of cultural competence in clinical supervision and suggest ways to improve the working alliance.

Social justice in clinical supervision

As mental health professionals, we are simultaneously ethically committed to the people we treat and to the well-being of society as a whole. Similarly, supervisors have a responsibility to respect the worldviews of their supervisees and their supervisees' clients, regardless of how much they might differ from their own. One of the guiding principles of social work, as stated in the profession's code of ethics, is to promote sensitivity to and knowledge about oppression and cultural and ethnic diversity, and to ensure access to needed information, services, and resources (National Association of Social Workers, 2015).

Similar guidelines are offered by the American Psychological Association (2019). This involves looking at how supervisors' and supervisees' own biases and assumptions may affect supervision and the supervisory relationship. The most recent edition of the APA's guidelines acknowledges that particular attention should be paid to race and ethnicity. Further, supervisors should be aware of their "positionality," which is defined by the APA as one's position or place in the racial and sociocultural hierarchy. This includes reflecting on the ways in which our statuses affect power dynamics and contribute to factors such as privilege and oppression. One way to enhance awareness, the APA suggests, is to participate in group activities such as workshops or professional interest groups that involve discussions of societal structures and related factors like oppression. Similarly, the United Kingdom Council for Psychotherapy (2018) explicitly states its commitment to addressing issues such as discrimination, prejudice, and oppression, and outlines how these factors may impact mental health professionals and their clients.

As we are currently witnessing a cultural shift taking place in the wake of the Black Lives Matter movement against anti-Black racism, supervisors and their supervisees are faced with a quandary in terms of striking a balance between therapeutic neutrality and social justice. When we observe instances of racism in the treatment room or in the supervisory hour, is it irresponsible for us (as either therapists or supervisors) to remain silent? How do we address the elephant in the room while at the same time maintaining a safe therapeutic holding environment? How can supervisors maintain a safe space and a positive supervisory working alliance while also remaining committed to social justice? How do we address these complex and often uncomfortable dynamics?

Surprisingly, our literature review did not reveal many studies that explored social justice in the context of supervision. The majority of the studies that touched on social justice practices looked at those that could be implemented in a therapeutic setting and then replicated in supervision. Kahn and Monk (2017) explored the use of narrative therapy as a tool to promote a social justice perspective in supervision. Narrative therapy looks at the stories that people create about themselves, others, and the world around them. When these narratives are negative and harmful to one's sense of self, narrative therapy aims to change them to healthier ones. Applied in a political context, supervisors (and therefore therapists) should aim to explore a client's beliefs and values that perpetuate oppression (like racism, for example) and help the client understand how those beliefs—often instilled by sociopolitical influences—negatively affect their life directly. In other words, rather than trying to change a societal outcome, therapists and supervisors should aim to change the actual conditions of their clients' lives. Speaking to the seemingly contrasting stances of therapeutic neutrality and the insertion of political matters in supervision, Kahn and Monk explained that supervisors and mental health professionals should take a political stand against the oppressive influences that impact clients' lives. They further stated that injustice can be understood as the direct result of power's covert manifestation. For example, the supervision encounter can in turn be seen as an opportunity for creating social change.

Asakura and Maurer (2018, p. 289) described supervision as "an optimal space within which clinicians can develop knowledge and skills to attend to the issues related to social justice in their practice." In their review of the literature, they identified three key elements to operationally define socially just clinical supervision: (1) attending to power relations in a supervisory dyad; (2) promoting the supervisee's reflective practice; and (3) cultivating advocacy skills among supervisees (Asakura & Maurer, 2018, p. 290). Reflective practice, or "the use of self," is an essential tool for clinicians and supervisors to use to gain further insight into the patient, such as by paying attention to unconscious reactions to clinical material. As it relates to social justice, the practice of reflection also includes the supervisor's and supervisee's awareness of sociocultural factors, such as privilege and oppression, and how these factors may impact the supervisee and the client and their supervisory and therapeutic relationships. Ongoing awareness and discussion of these factors, according to Asakura and Maurer (2018, p. 291), are "essential in facilitating the supervisees' abilities to understand the interplay between the client issues and larger social structures and challenging the supervisee's own biases and stereotypes."

Supervisors can play a major role in the incorporation of social justice into the therapeutic setting as well as into the mental health profession. Assuming that supervisors have examined their own internal cultural and racial biases, they should be able to help their supervisees do the same. Safety is vital in establishing a strong supervisory working alliance, which makes it a prerequisite for establishing effective supervision that promotes social justice. In order to gain a better understanding of supervisees' experiences of safe supervision, ChenFeng et al. (2017) interviewed multiple supervisees from various cultures. Based on these interviews, the authors identified the following three variables in fostering safety and social justice in the supervisory relationship:

1 *Supervisor authenticity and vulnerability.* Through supervisors' self-disclosure and acknowledgment of their positionality, supervisees felt

comfortable discussing issues of diversity, such as when a supervisor shared their own experiences with racism or discrimination.

2 *Validation of supervisees' experience.* Supervisees felt heard and seen for who they were, including their social identity, when their supervisors were open to learning about their experiences and backgrounds, as well as being open to feedback.
3 *Witnessing supervisor's empathy and compassion.* Interestingly, another common element among supervisees was their observation of their supervisor's behavior outside of supervision, such as their supervisor's ability to empathize with their clients. The main point is that supervisors must be open to receiving honest feedback from their supervisees in order for social justice to be advanced and for supervision to feel safe. Promoting a sense of safety and social justice within the supervisory relationship will affect the supervisee's work and therefore promote safety and social justice in the lives of their clients.

In response to the dearth of research, Fickling et al. (2019) looked at the Multicultural and Social Justice Counseling Competencies (MSJCC) model (Ratts et al., 2016) as it applies to clinical supervision. The MSJCC model was designed to help practitioners understand racial and other sociocultural dynamics. By applying this model to supervision, the authors aimed to identify a framework that supervisors can use to further their multicultural and social justice competencies. Supervisors could then model this framework with their supervisees, who, in turn, may apply it to their work with clients. The four developmental domains of the MSJCC model that the authors suggested applying to supervision include: (1) supervisor's self-awareness of their racial and cultural identity; (2) awareness of the supervisee's worldview and identity; (3) the supervisory relationship; and (4) supervision and advocacy interventions. The authors noted that the lack of research in the fourth domain as it applies specifically to supervision calls for practitioners and researchers to identify social justice competencies addressing privilege, oppression, and power dynamics in the supervisory relationship.

Cultural competence in cross-cultural supervision

Cultural competence is significant in the clinical supervision process. Although the literature around cultural competence in the field of counseling has grown exponentially in the last decade or so, this has unfortunately not been extended to clinical supervision (Peters, 2017; Wilcox et al., 2020). For example, how supervisors and supervisees navigate their own different cultural backgrounds and language barriers and how this affects the supervision process and the supervisory working alliance has only partially been answered through research. Therefore, it is necessary to understand how cultural competence affects supervision and the multiple variables that come into play when the supervisor and the supervisee are from different cultural backgrounds.

Watkins and Milne (2014, p. 14) defined cultural competence as "the ability to work effectively with people with distinctive qualities, including their country, ethnicity and culture." Simply put, cultural competence is being sensitive to the fact that what may be considered unusual in one's own culture could be commonplace in another. It is the assurance that we do not pathologize behaviors or values simply because they do not align with our own.

As mental health clinicians, we will inevitably work with individuals from different backgrounds, cultures, ethnicities, and religions than our own. Most if not all educational training prepares students to provide culturally competent treatment. For example, the American Psychological Association (2019) requires multicultural training in all of its accredited professional psychology programs. Nevertheless, we wonder how prominent this topic is in the training and education of supervisors, particularly when we emphasize the intersection between clinical supervision and culturally competent treatment (Estrada, 2018).

There is a need to recognize diversity within the supervision triad, not only between supervisor and supervisee but also between therapist (supervisee) and patient. While it is the task of the supervisor to be sensitive to multicultural issues within the supervisor–supervisee relationship, it is also important to teach supervisees how such factors impact the therapeutic relationship. By considering cultural variables within the supervisory relationship, the supervisor inadvertently teaches the supervisee to consider how these variables impact the patient's inner life and the therapeutic relationship. It also impacts the supervisee's conceptualization of the patient when presented in supervision (Chopra, 2013). Both the supervisor and the supervisee in cross-cultural supervision must figure out how to navigate their different social mores and values and overcome language barriers and other clashes of cultural norms that impact supervision and the supervisory relationship.

Ancis and Marshall (2010) explained that multicultural supervision occurs when both the supervisor and the supervisee consider an array of cultural matters involving them and/or their clients from diverse backgrounds. The authors interviewed four psychology graduate students about their experiences in supervision, specifically asking about the dynamic with their supervisors when facilitating cross-cultural conversations. They found that successful multicultural supervision experiences were connected to supervisors who were actively exploring multicultural issues with the goal of increasing their understanding of their clients and of themselves, and to supervisors who were aware of their own cultural backgrounds, experiences, and biases—or those who spoke openly about not knowing enough about the multicultural elements of supervision.

Lee (2018) reviewed the literature on the supervision of international supervisees and explained that the major barriers in cross-cultural supervision are: (1) acculturation and cultural difference; (2) language barriers; (3) social isolation; (4) cultural perceptions of the profession and transferability; and (5) multicultural discussions. The author recommended that supervisees discuss these barriers with their supervisors to ensure that supervisors are aware of the challenges that their supervisees experience outside of supervision and within the supervisory relationship. Lee's findings reflect the evidence we gathered through our conversations with supervisees from diverse cultures. Specifically, we learned that traditional supervision is not as effective for an analyst in training who is treating patients and writing a process recording in the Korean language, translating it into English, and receiving supervision in English. This can be a grueling process that can potentially compromise the authenticity of the case presentation, and to some degree the effectiveness of the supervisory hour. The supervisor's awareness of these details is the key to improving the effectiveness of culturally competent supervision.

McKinley (2019) explored the best practices for supervising international students by using two case vignettes from the experiences of international supervisees in a clinical psychology program based in the United States. Findings from this inquiry showed that it is pivotal for the supervisor to be aware of their own cultural identity in order to develop multicultural supervision competencies. Supervisors who feel inadequate or uncomfortable addressing cultural issues may choose to ignore or fail to address them in their discussions with supervisees, and therefore compromise the alliance. McKinley also elaborated on the supervisor's need to be open to cultural humility, which is the ability to maintain an interpersonal stance of openness to others' cultural identities.

In a recent qualitative study with 14 supervisors, Zoricelis (2019) explored the interactions that took place in supervision sessions that led to the integration or avoidance of multicultural conversations. An analysis of the data using grounded theory revealed three themes: (1) integration of multicultural topics and materials in the supervisory meetings; (2) competent multicultural supervisor who teaches, implements, and practices intentionality of integration of cultural discussions; and (3) competent multicultural supervision process to integrate cultural discussions. Zoricelis added that once the intention to integrate multicultural topics exists, there are additional mediators to promote multicultural supervision, such as the supervisory relationship, the supervisor's responsibility, and the supervisor's personal and professional characteristics. In terms of holding multicultural discussions in supervision, a supervisor should be able to assess their supervisee's readiness to talk about multicultural topics and then teach them, integrate them, and encourage supervisees to speak about them.

The Competent Multicultural Counseling Supervision model is also supported by previous work. Tohidian and Quek (2017) conducted a qualitative meta-analysis (n = 24) to learn about supervisory practices with an emphasis on diversity. Their findings revealed the presence of six meta-categories: (1) supervisor's multicultural stances; (2) supervisee's multicultural encounters; (3) competency-based content in supervision; (4) processes surrounding multicultural supervision; (5) culturally attuned interventions; and (6) multicultural supervisory alliance. The results of their study mainly focused on supervisors, emphasizing that in multicultural supervision, the supervisor is ultimately responsible for developing the supervisee's multicultural competence by integrating discussions about cultural competence. They highlighted that multicultural supervision is also related to the supervisee's multicultural encounters and their willingness to discuss these encounters with their supervisor. This prompts us to look at effective culturally competent supervision from the supervisee's perspective.

Finally, Tsui et al. (2014) stressed the need to consider both cross-cultural and "intracultural" supervision in culturally competent supervision, referring to paying attention not only to dominant cultures but also to the indigenous and minority populations within a country or region. They recommended that all supervisors consider the following guiding principles when working cross-culturally:

- The political context: The structural differentiation, class differences, and political ideologies of the supervisee and the supervisor.
- The cultural context: The values, norms, rituals, and customs of the social environment.
- The organizational context: The occupational hierarchy, use of supervisory authority, and decision-making in the process of clinical supervision.
- Professional practices: The clinical expertise, professional roles, staff participation, learning process, and supervisory interaction.
- Personal characteristics: The personal background and uniqueness of individual supervisees and supervisors, e.g., their age, gender, race, religion, and physical characteristics.

Supervisees' perceptions of cultural competence in cross-cultural supervision

Supervisors are ultimately responsible for developing the supervisee's multicultural competence by integrating discussions about cultural competence in their supervision sessions. Responsive therapy falls on supervisors as the more experienced members of the profession (Chang & Chang, 2016; Estrada, 2018; Inman, 2006). In fact, the cross-cultural supervisory relationship is positively correlated with the supervisor's genuine interest in other cultures, their ability to create a sense of safety so that cultural differences can be discussed, and their ability to foster an environment in which supervisees feel comfortable with self-disclosure (Chopra, 2013). According to Yee (2018), these qualities may be even more important than the supervisor's actual degree of competence in cross-cultural supervision.

In contrast, when supervisees perceive their supervisors to be lacking in multicultural sensitivity, they experience the supervisory process as ineffective. In addition to a lack of awareness of cultural differences, unintentional racism, overemphasizing cultural factors to explain psychological difficulties, and an inability to give valuable feedback may hinder the development of a supervisory safe space and thereby sabotage the working alliance (Chopra, 2013; Peters, 2017).

In response to the lack of research on the perspectives of supervisees, Hutman and Ellis (2020) looked at supervisees' nondisclosure and its variables related to multicultural competence. Using data from 221 mental health supervisees in training, the authors found an inverse correlation between supervisees' perceptions of their supervisors' multicultural competence and their tendency to withhold information related to both the supervision and to the clinical case material. Further, they found the supervisory working alliance to be a mediating factor between supervisees' nondisclosure and supervisors' cultural competence. The authors attributed these findings to the prevalence of a hierarchical structure in supervision and supervisees' concerns about being judged negatively by their supervisors. These findings support the notion that supervisors who are multiculturally competent foster an environment that is conducive to developing a more authentic supervisory relationship and therefore leads to effective supervision.

The idea of cultural humility, which refers to the supervisor's attentiveness to cultural differences in the supervisory relationship, makes a significant contribution to multicultural supervision when the supervisor is ready to engage in multicultural conversations and learn alongside their supervisee about their different cultural backgrounds and worldviews (Watkins et al., 2019). Cook et al. (2020) surveyed 101 post-master's counseling supervisees to assess the connection between the cultural humility of the supervisor and intentional nondisclosure of the supervisee. Using 21 questions from the Cultural Humility Scale (supervision version), they found that 20 percent of supervisees' intentional nondisclosure could be explained by their perceptions of their supervisors' level of cultural humility. Their study was the first to empirically assess how cultural humility impacts the supervisory relationship.

Moreover, King et al. (2020) surveyed 67 master's counseling students and their supervisors about multicultural orientation (MCO) functions in supervision. To collect data, the authors used various scales, such as the Supervisee Cultural Awareness Scale, the MCO adapted scale, the Cultural Humility Scale, four questions about cultural missed opportunities, cultural behavior scales, and the Working Alliance Inventory/Supervision. The results showed that supervisor cultural humility and missed opportunities to discuss culture predicted the supervisory working alliance but did not directly affect it. King et al. have recommended that in order to increase effective multicultural supervision and increase supervisees' cultural awareness, supervisors should focus on suggesting interventions that demonstrate MCO in supervision.

Similarly, Estrada (2018) has encouraged supervisors to engage their supervisees in a reflection on and discussion of supervisees' own cultural identities and their influence on supervision. The author recommended cultural genograms as one example of a practical tool that can be used by supervisors to increase their supervisees' awareness of the impact of culture. Such concrete tools should be used in tandem with the emotional processing of supervisees' own cultural histories; for example, when working with supervisees from minority groups, they should explore the history of the societal oppression of those groups. Speaking to the reciprocal nature of the supervisory relationship, Estrada added that it is also the responsibility of supervisees to engage in furthering their own knowledge and to strive to develop their cultural sensitivity and responsiveness.

Cross-cultural supervision between Western and Asian cultures

Psychological counseling in its contemporary format has only been implemented in most Asian countries within the last 40 years. Since these countries' current mental health practices and conventions are based on those that were mainly imported from the West, their practitioners need to have access to qualified supervisors on opposite sides of the world.

Although clinical supervision as a practice domain has not yet been formally established in countries such as China, awareness of the necessity of supervision is rapidly growing within the mental health community there (Duan et al., 2019; Scharff, 2016). Between 2002 and 2006, in response to the great need for Chinese students, psychologists, psychiatrists, and counselors to have access to supervisors, the China American Psychoanalytic Alliance (CAPA) was established as a volunteer organization to recruit and assign supervisors from the United States and other Western countries to work with Chinese mental health professionals. Snyder described the inspiration for CAPA as follows:

> Friends and colleagues in the U.S. provided supervision on the phone and by e-mail. Finally, one man asked me to find an analyst for him. I said, "But, there are no analysts in China." He said, "What about Skype?" I said, "What is Skype?" and thus, CAPA was born.
>
> (Snyder, 2020, p. 17)

CAPA provides a great example of cross-cultural systematic training and psychoanalytic psychotherapy supervision. Campbell (2020) has provided insight into the supervisory relationship between an American supervisor and a Chinese supervisee by highlighting the need for supervisees to learn how to be a supervisee, present a case, and address affect and its expression in relation to language barriers. He concluded that this cultural adjustment can be made easier when there are conversations about boundaries and expectations as well as specific guidelines or a common point of reference, which are provided by CAPA.

Western supervisors working cross-culturally with supervisees from Asia must consider the many fundamental differences that exist between them in terms of their cultural values. These include differences between collectivist versus individualist societies, independence versus interdependence, and social equality versus a hierarchical system. Perhaps most importantly, power differentials within these supervisory relationships must be explored. In contrast to individualistic societies, such as those found in Europe and North America, where individual opinions and self-expression are prioritized (Yee, 2018), collectivist societies, such as those found in Asia, place a greater value on the group over the individual. One of the ways this may manifest among supervisees from Asian countries is through their communication style, which is likely to be more indirect and non-confrontational, and they may have difficulty expressing feelings of anger. A supervisor who is unaware of these cultural values may judge this behavior negatively rather than understand it as a cultural norm perpetuated by the desire to maintain social harmony. Additionally, a supervisor who is more direct and encourages self-expression may cause some discomfort for the supervisee who is not used to it (Yee, 2018).

In Chapter 4, a supervisee living in China and studying with CAPA describes the initial tension she felt when she began remote supervision with her American supervisor. As a student raised in China, her education had been profoundly influenced by neo-Confucianism, which prioritizes respect for authority and therefore does not allow for much discussion to take place or for the supervisee to diverge from the supervisor. This tension manifested in her following some of her supervisor's suggestions, although she silently disagreed with them. Her supervisor, aware of the cultural factors at play, fostered a supervisory relationship based on equality by reassuring her of her autonomy and telling her that she did not have to accept every suggestion that the supervisor made. This offers a clear example of cultural competence in action.

Another example of an organization designed to implement formal supervision training in Asia is the Korean Association of Psychoanalysis (KAPA), a component of the International Psychoanalytic Association (IPA). Formed in response to the lack of psychoanalysts in the country, it is composed of a formal study group in which IPA-recognized analysts—either partly or fully trained in the United States—are invited to supervise Korean analysts in training (Jeong, 2019). In Chapter 5, a Korean supervisee describes his experience as a member of KAPA. In particular, he describes being remotely supervised by an American supervisor. During one supervision session in particular, as he was presenting his Korean patient to his supervisor, he explained to her the concept of the Chinese zodiac. In the Chinese zodiac, one's birth year is represented by an animal that carries a special meaning about the person's fate. Discussing this cultural concept with his supervisor who had been previously unfamiliar with it gave both of them fresh insight into the inner life of the presented patient. Similar examples can be found throughout the chapters in this book.

Son et al. (2013) have found that supervisees from South Korea tend to view their supervisors as high-ranking authorities, and are thus less likely to disclose their thoughts and feelings to them. Needless to say, these factors pose a challenge to the building of the supervisory working alliance, and therefore must be taken into consideration by supervisors. According to Bang and Park (2009, p. 1069):

> Sharing of vulnerabilities clashes with the cultural emphasis on face-saving that pervades the norms regarding interpersonal relationships in Korean culture. To save face, Korean supervisees may put a great deal of pressure on themselves to be perfect and to find "the right answer" in their clinical work. It would have a normalizing effect on the supervisee if the supervisor explained that it is impossible not to make any mistakes in clinical work, shared clinical mistakes the supervisor made in his or her clinical work, and told the supervisee how he or she recovered from those mistakes.

The authors suggested that supervisors should exhibit sensitivity toward their supervisees' efforts to ask for help by asking the supervisee what they have done so far to address their concerns before providing feedback to the supervisee. The authors also emphasized the need for supervisors to work toward disentangling supervisees' language proficiency from their clinical competency. Just as supervisees from Western cultures need trust, support, and mutual agreement within the supervisory relationship, so too do supervisees from Asian cultures. Therefore, supervisors from non-Asian cultures should remain attuned to these role conflicts and power dynamics and their effects on the supervisory working alliance.

Conclusions

If we are to be effective clinicians, we must be as competent in our understanding of cultural differences as we are in our knowledge of individual psychology. It would stand to reason that the same should be applied to supervisors. It is true that it is the responsibility of supervisors to become educated in order to effectively supervise clinicians from diverse backgrounds who will undoubtedly also be working with patients from backgrounds different from their own. Nevertheless, this may not always be the case, and supervisors are not always aware of significant differences that affect the work. It is important for us to point out that effective culturally competent supervision also depends on the supervisee, who should advocate for a culturally diverse learning experience in supervision.

While there is a growing body of literature on social justice in counseling and clinical supervision, research that specifically looks at social justice factors from the perspective of the supervisee is lacking. Further exploration of supervisees' experiences would produce valuable material and contribute to the promotion of social justice in the profession.

Since factors such as race, ethnicity, and socio-economic background significantly influence the lives of our patients, the therapeutic relationship, and the treatment itself, they should not be taken lightly. The same sentiment ought to be applied to supervision. Supervision is an optimal space within which clinicians can develop the self-awareness, knowledge, and skills they need to attend to the issues related to cultural differences in their practices. Throughout this book are several examples demonstrating culturally competent supervision. In all of these cases, one of the most significant aspects of the supervisory relationship—the working alliance—will be presented as a primary determinant in shaping supervisees' perceptions of effective supervision as it relates to cultural competence.

References

Akkurt, M. N., Ng, K. M., & Kolbert, J. (2018). Multicultural discussion as a moderator of counseling supervision-related constructs. *International Journal for the Advancement of Counselling*, 40(4), 455–468.

American Psychological Association. (2019). *Race and ethnicity guidelines in psychology: Promoting responsiveness and equity.* www.apa.org/about/policy/race-and-ethnicity-in-psychology.pdf.

Ancis, J., & Marshall, D. (2010). Using a multicultural framework to assess supervisees' perceptions of culturally competent supervision. *Journal of Counseling and Development*, 88(3), 277–284.

Asakura, K., & Maurer, K. (2018). Attending to social justice in clinical social work: Supervision as a pedagogical space. *Clinical Social Work Journal*, 46(4), 289–297. doi:10.1007/s10615-018-0667-4.

Bang, K., & Park, J. (2009). Korean supervisors' experiences in clinical supervision. *The Counseling Psychologist*, 37(8), 1042–1075.

Campbell, T. W. (2020). CAPA supervision. *Psychoanalytic Inquiry*, 40(1), 38–45.

Chang, S., & Chang, S. S. (2016). A study on psychotherapy supervisor's education and training components. *Journal of the Korea Contents Association*, 16(4), 488–502.

ChenFeng, J., Castronova, M., & Zimmerman, T. (2017). Safety and social justice in the supervisory relationship. In R. Allan & S. Singh Poulsen (Eds.), *Creating cultural safety in couple and family therapy* (pp. 43–56). Springer.

Chopra, T. (2013). All supervision is multicultural: A review of literature on the need for multicultural supervision in counseling. *Psychological Studies*, 58(3), 335–338.

Cook, R. M., Jones, C. T., & Welfare, L. E. (2020). Supervisor cultural humility predicts intentional nondisclosure by post-master's counselors. *Counselor Education and Supervision*, 59(2), 160–167.

Duan, C., Falender, C., Goodyear, R., Qian, M., Jia, X., & Jiang, G. (2019). Telesupervision-of-supervision across national boundaries: United States and China. *Journal of Clinical Psychology*, 75(2), 302–312.

Estrada, D. (2018). Training and supervision across disciplines to engage in cross-cultural competence and responsiveness: Counseling and family therapy. In S. Singh Poulsen & R. Allan (Eds.), *Cross-cultural responsiveness and systemic therapy* (pp. 101–117). Springer.

Fickling, M. J., Tangen, J. L., Graden, M. W., & Grays, D. (2019). Multicultural and social justice competence in clinical supervision. *Counselor Education and Supervision*, 58(4), 309–316.

Hird, J. S., Cavalieri, C. E., Dulko, J. P., Felice, A. A., & Ho, T. A. (2001). Visions and realities: Supervisee perspectives of multicultural supervision. *Journal of Multicultural Counseling and Development*, 29(2), 114–130.

Hutman, H., & Ellis, M. V. (2020). Supervisee nondisclosure in clinical supervision: Cultural and relational considerations. *Training and Education in Professional Psychology*, 14(4), 308–315. doi:10.1037/tep0000290.

Inman, A. G. (2006). Supervisor multicultural competence and its relation to supervisory process and outcome. *Journal of Marital and Family Therapy*, 32(1), 73–85.

Jeong, D. U. (2019). The Korean psychoanalytic movement and the IPA (1980–2010). In P. Loewenberg & N. L. Thompson (Eds.). *100 years of the IPA: The centenary history of the International Psychoanalytical Association, 1910–2010: Evolution and change* (pp. 404–411). Karnac.

Kahn, S. Z., & Monk, G. (2017). Narrative supervision as a social justice practice. *Journal of Systemic Therapies*, 36(1), 7–25.

King, K. M., Borders, L. D., & Jones, C. T. (2020). Multicultural orientation in clinical supervision: Examining impact through dyadic data. *The Clinical Supervisor*, 39(1), 1–24. doi:10.1080/07325223.2020.1763223.

Lee, A. (2018). Clinical supervision of international supervisees: Suggestions for multicultural supervision. *International Journal for the Advancement of Counselling*, 40(1), 60–71.

McKinley, M. T. (2019). Supervising the sojourner: Multicultural supervision of international students. *Training and Education in Professional Psychology*, 13(3), 174–179. doi:10.1037/tep0000269.

National Association of Social Workers. (2015). *Code of ethics*. www.socialworkers.org/pubs/code/code.asp.

Peters, H. C. (2017). Multicultural complexity: An intersectional lens for clinical supervision. *International Journal for the Advancement of Counselling*, 39, 176–187.

Ratts, M. J., Singh, A. A., Nassar-McMillan, S., Butler, S. K., & McCullough, J. R. (2016). Multicultural and social justice counseling competencies: Guidelines for the counseling profession. *Journal of Multicultural Counseling and Development*, 44(1), 28–48.

Scharff, D. E. (2016). Psychoanalysis in China: An essay on the recent literature in English. *Psychoanalytic Quarterly*, 85(4), 1037–1067. doi:10.1002/psaq.12121.

Snyder, E. W. (2020). The history of CAPA. *Psychoanalytic Inquiry*, 40(1), 16–29.

Son, E., Ellis, M. V., & Yoo, S.-K. (2013). Clinical supervision in South Korea and the United States: A comparative descriptive study. *The Counseling Psychologist*, 41(1), 48–65.

Tohidian, N. B., & Quek, K. M. T. (2017). Processes that inform multicultural supervision: A qualitative meta-analysis. *Journal of Marital and Family Therapy*, 43(4), 573–590.

Tsui, M., O'Donoghue, K., & Ng, A. K. T. (2014). Culturally-competent and diversity-sensitive clinical supervision: An international perspective. In C. E.Watkins, Jr., & D. L. Milne (Eds.), *Wiley international handbook of clinical supervision* (pp. 238–254). Wiley.

United Kingdom Council for Psychotherapy. (2018). *Practice guidelines for supervisors*. www.psychotherapy.org.uk/wp-content/uploads/2019/01/UKCP-Practice-Guidelines-for-Supervisors-2018.pdf.

Watkins, C. E., Hook, J. N., Mosher, D. K., & Callahan, J. L. (2019). Humility in clinical supervision: Fundamental, foundational, and transformational. *The Clinical Supervisor*, 38(1), 58–78.

Watkins, C. E., Jr., & Milne, D. L. (Eds.). (2014). *The Wiley international handbook of clinical supervision*. Wiley.

Wilcox, M. M., Franks, D. N., Taylor, T. O., Monceaux, C. P., & Harris, K. (2020). Who's multiculturally competent? Everybody and nobody: A multimethod examination. *The Counseling Psychologist*, 48(4), 466–497.

Yee, T. (2018). Supervising East Asian international students: Incorporating culturally responsive supervision into the integrated developmental model. *The Clinical Supervisor*, 37(2), 298–312.

Zoricelis, D. (2019). *Integrating multicultural discussions in counseling supervision: A grounded theory study* (Publication No. 2116) [Doctoral dissertation, Liberty University]. Scholars Crossing, the institutional repository of Liberty University. https://digitalcommons.liberty.edu/doctoral/2116.

Chapter 4

Effective supervision despite cultural and theoretical differences

Ruiqi Tian

Preface

I have always had a genuine interest in supervision. I am a supervisor myself, and I conduct a fair amount of research focused on the working alliance between supervisors and supervisees, specifically in China, which is where I live and where there is a small number of qualified supervisors and a dearth of academic training and concrete guidelines for clinical supervision. I was lucky to connect with Dr. Barbara Stimmel when she worked with the China American Psychoanalytic Alliance (CAPA) as a faculty member and supervisor. My relationship with her as her supervisee has continued to this day. I believe that the quality of supervision matters, and my work with Dr. Stimmel has certainly reinforced that belief.

I feel refreshed and renewed after almost every supervision session with Dr. Stimmel. She helps me clarify a lot of my confusion in the analytic work, which in turn enables me to fully enjoy and be confident in my work with clients. Through supervision sessions with Dr. Stimmel, I have developed an ability to treat my clients more naturally—free of judgment or fear of making mistakes. I am able to understand their journeys in a more empathetic way and without getting overly involved. Consequently, my clients are able to accept themselves better, feel less anxious about facing their traumas and pains, and overcome conflicts. Indirectly, my supervisees also benefit from my relationship with Dr. Stimmel. They are able to more easily let go of their own anxieties and excessive pursuits of their narcissistic needs, and thus gradually help their clients tolerate the ups and downs of life.

When I was invited by Liat and Allison to contribute to this book, it was hard to believe that my feelings of appreciation for Dr. Stimmel and my gains from our work together were not unique to me but were also shared by so many of her other supervisees from around the world. Liat and Allison invited us—the supervisees of Dr. Stimmel—to think more deeply and systematically about our experiences and to gain a better understanding of the supervision process by contributing to this book.

Dr. Stimmel is my fourth individual supervisor. Before I met her, I had been supervised by three other supervisors once a week for five years. All of them were excellent psychoanalysts and supervisors, and each furthered my professional development in different ways. However, it was only through my work with Dr. Stimmel that I was able to experience deeply the beauty of therapeutic work and fully enjoy the supervision process—both as a supervisor and as a supervisee. I would like to thank Liat and Allison for giving me this opportunity to share my experience.

Cultural differences

Despite our significant cultural, training, and theoretical differences, I have gained a lot from Dr. Stimmel's supervision. Since the Han Dynasty (202 BCE–220 CE), Chinese feudal rulers have followed Dong Zhongshu's neo-Confucian philosophy advocating the divine right of kings, with the sovereign holding absolute power and requiring total submission to his authority. Neo-Confucianism has long influenced teacher–student relationships in China as well. Whatever the teacher says, the student must accept, and they must not challenge that hierarchy. As a result, Chinese students have traditionally had limited opportunities to develop their critical thinking skills or even discuss differences in opinion. Although this authoritarian influence pervaded Chinese culture well into the twentieth century, China's educational system has undergone revolution and reform in recent decades. These cultural and philosophical shifts have led both teaching and supervision to be profoundly influenced by neo-Confucianism and postmodern thought today.

The neo-Confucian approach to the teacher–student relationship requires the student to respect the teacher and value their teaching, which leaves little room for discussion, divergence, or dissent. By contrast, postmodernism advocates subverting authority and welcomes intellectual debate, which conflicts with the traditional Chinese teacher–student dyad. Dr. Stimmel, who had never been to China, demonstrated a typical American postmodern approach to supervision when we began. She would tell me what she thought and advise me simply and directly. The conflicting influences of my educational training and her way of thinking made me doubt the validity of Dr. Stimmel's clinical suggestions at the beginning of our supervisory relationship. However, I still followed her advice—despite not quite understanding the clinical meaning behind it—because I had been taught to respect my teachers. Although I did not quite agree with her suggestions when we spoke about a client I presented, I felt an overwhelming urge to obey her—mainly out of cultural habit and not necessarily because I believed in what she was saying. Later, that all changed; the client's reaction to my new approach (which was based on Dr. Stimmel's suggestions) made me realize that she had been right, and I then began to develop real trust in her.

For example, I once spoke with Dr. Stimmel about a client who had to travel more than two hours to see me in person; to save on travel time, we conducted video sessions instead.[1] Dr. Stimmel first explored the client's realistic reasons for wanting to conduct the supervision over video instead of physically coming to the office and running the risk of being late. She also proposed that this may have connected to the client's resistance. She may have been avoiding the negative feelings associated with arriving late or facing the consequences thereof. As a result, the resistance was solved by conducting video sessions to eliminate the conscious and unconscious reasons behind the client's failure to arrive at sessions on time.

Dr. Stimmel firmly suggested that I revert to face-to-face sessions with this client so I could have a better chance of addressing her resistance. But I fully identified with the client and did not see the difference between video sessions and face-to-face sessions. It seemed impractical for the client to travel more than two hours just to see me, so why did Dr. Stimmel insist that she needed to come to the office?

Dr. Stimmel provided firm and confident advice but reinforced that our relationship was based on equality and mutual respect by reassuring me that she was only making a suggestion and not forcing me to take it up. Yet, to show respect for my teacher (as I was used to doing), I recommended that the client see me in person, even though I strongly identified with her struggle to do so. I even felt a little angry with Dr. Stimmel, just as my client was angry with me when we both submitted to our respective authority figures.

In this case, it all worked out in a very positive way. I followed Dr. Stimmel's guidance to help the client transition from video to face-to-face sessions; in return, this helped the client tell me about her relational pattern with persecutory authority. This experience made me reflect not only on the dynamic between the client and me but also on cultural differences when communicating with an authority figure by thinking about both my habit and my client's habit of submitting to authority.

Differences between theoretical schools

There are not only cultural differences between Dr. Stimmel and me, but also differences in our theoretical orientations. I am trained as a counseling psychologist, and am currently working as a school counselor and as a therapist in private practice. I am engaged in university teaching, research, and supervision. Over the years, I have studied many therapeutic approaches, such as cognitive behavioral therapy (CBT), family therapy, hypnotherapy, sandplay therapy, Gestalt therapy, painting therapy, etc. I currently use more CBT for my short-term clients in the university, and, as a supervisor, I use more of a competency model than a pure psychoanalytic supervisory model.

When I began my studies in an intensive psychodynamic program in 2010, I started to receive systematic training in psychodynamic therapy. While I am supervised by Dr. Stimmel and am also in analysis, I have no intention of becoming a psychoanalyst. Psychoanalysis influences the way I think, but it is not my specialty. I use a cross-school perspective in my therapeutic work; and, within psychoanalysis, I am interested in relational psychoanalysis, whereas Dr. Stimmel comes from a Freudian school of thought. When I began supervision with her, I worried that our very different theoretical approaches would create some tension between us.

Dr. Stimmel became my supervisor by chance. The training program assigned her as my individual supervisor during Year 4 of my studies, and I was not familiar with her before we met. In our first meeting, I talked about my theoretical orientation and professional plans and goals. Dr. Stimmel then suggested that it might be better if I asked the program to reassign me to a supervisor from a relational school of thought instead. Although I knew nothing about her, I dismissed her suggestion. Her overall tone conveyed a professional confidence and firmness which intrigued me and made me want to learn more about what she had to offer. The subsequent two and a half years of supervision proved that I had made the correct decision despite our cultural and theoretical differences, and I discovered that there are other more critical factors that determine the success of supervision, which I will discuss below.

Factors promoting good supervisory relationships

I have found that the following factors promote the effectiveness of the supervisory relationship: (1) the realness of the supervisor; (2) the professional competence of the supervisor; (3) the high sense of self-regard and self-efficacy of the supervisor; (4) the respect of the supervisor for the supervisee; and (5) the strong emotional bond or attachment in the supervisory dyad.

The realness of the supervisor

Dr. Stimmel's realness anchors our supervisory relationship. In the more than two years that I have spent under her supervision, she has not deliberately maintained any facades—she just behaves as herself. This sense of authenticity makes me feel stable and confident. However, this supervisory relationship differs from my past experiences. I once had a supervisor from whom I also learned a lot and to whom I felt grateful, but I could hardly sense her authenticity and consistency. She was even defensive (in my eyes), so that I was not satisfied with her—and I even felt a little angry toward her. I once made an Excel table to record the frequency of her lateness, early departure, number of telephone calls she answered during supervision, and number of sessions she forgot.

In traditional Chinese culture, we are taught to respect our teachers. Even now, when we question our mentors, it is only with regard to diverging opinions on intellectual concepts; for fear of offending and disrespecting them, we do not question the mentors themselves. However, my dissatisfaction with that particular supervisor grew until one day I gathered the courage to say to her, "Even though you always explain why you have arrived late and left early and answered the phone during supervisory sessions, it still makes me feel uncomfortable in our supervision, which reduces the effectiveness of our supervision." She replied that my reaction was based on the parallel process and combined it with my clinical case to illustrate her point. I admitted that for my client, the authority in her head was cruel and indifferent, and she was full of anger at authority. But my dissatisfaction with my supervisor was real, and I rejected the claim that the parallel process could explain every aspect of the supervisory relationship. My former supervisor's explanation made me realize that she was defensive, which made me even more angry. I could only truly identify that once I entered into supervision with Dr. Stimmel and presented the same case. I have never had a similar dissatisfaction with Dr. Stimmel; she has never been defensive and is always curious to know my thoughts.

I believe that what made me uncomfortable in my previous supervisory experience was not the supervisor's behavior per se, but her defensive and insincere attitude toward our relationship. She was not an authentic person to me, and we failed to establish a mutually trusting supervisory relationship. By contrast, Dr. Stimmel's authenticity has allowed us to establish a real relationship in which I have been able to process and tolerate sometimes negative emotions. Gelso and Carter (1985) claimed that the therapeutic relationship consists of the real relationship, transference configuration relationships, and the working alliance. This is also true for the supervisory relationship. Real relationships can break down supervisees' negative transference to their supervisors and build a stronger working alliance. As a result, the supervisory dyad can better focus on the supervisee's cases rather than the transference between them.

My need for a supervisor who is a "real person" links back to my traditional Chinese culture and the Taoist perspective. Taoism posits that simplicity and truth are at the root of all things, and that these will allow for the resolution of all kinds of conflict. From a Taoist perspective, realness facilitates effective supervision and supervisory relationships.

The professional competence of the supervisor

The second contributing factor to the effectiveness of our supervisory relationship is Dr. Stimmel's high academic competence as a supervisor. I have no intention here of offering a systematic and theoretical model of a supervisor's competence, but aim to simply provide evidence from my experiences with Dr. Stimmel. When I refer to competence, I mean having a deep understanding of clients, supervisees, and proper therapeutic and supervisory interventions. Dr. Stimmel has always been able to see the internal dynamics of the cases I report (even with little information), clarify my problems with the cases, and give me what I need—even when I do not know what that is.

An example of this is a supervision we had about a client I had been seeing for nearly eight years. My working alliance with the client was very stable. She took every consultation very seriously and tried her best to share with me everything going on in her mind. However, in one supervision session, Dr. Stimmel told me that from the narrative I had shared, she felt that my client was not being real and was not sincere with me. I was very surprised. It completely subverted my understanding of the case. I did not even think that I should doubt this hardworking and devoted client. At the beginning of our supervision, I questioned Dr. Stimmel's suggestions. Nonetheless, throughout the treatment and supervision processes, discoveries revealed in the treatments supported Dr. Stimmel's clinical wisdom. In this case, I firmly believe that Dr. Stimmel captured some of my blind spots—specifically, that I overidentified with the client without being aware of it.

As a result, I started to think back to the details of past sessions that I had had with this client, and I realized that when the client interacted with other people, there were indeed many differences between what she felt internally and what she expressed outwardly, but she always gave others the impression of sincerity. At the appropriate time, in subsequent sessions, I shared these findings with the client. She then acknowledged that she would select different themes and wordings in her communications based on her assessments of different people. In our treatment, she would choose the material that she thought I was interested in or that was consistent with my previous case conceptualizations. Although she had different feelings, she would only show me her anxiety and anger. During the process, she defended her hostility toward the outside world, including her hostility toward me. From her perspective, the outside world (especially sources of authority) was indifferent, cruel, and sadistic. Once we could explore this, the treatment deepened. Dr. Stimmel frequently helped me refresh my understanding of my cases and clarified my approach to subsequent interventions.

Dr. Stimmel's ability to accept clients and supervisees as they are, at that moment, and at their current level of understanding and analysis embodies the Taoist concept of allowing nature to take its course. For example, I once had a client who repeated her intergenerational trauma and was always attracted to the sadistic intimate relationship. One day, both of us missed our appointment for a session. In the next session, I invited her to reflect on how she felt about the fact that both of us had forgotten. She gave me a very concrete and realistic reasoning and reiterated her trust in me, saying that she did not have any negative feelings toward me. Later, she began to focus on what had happened in her life, and it seemed that our forgetting the session had never happened. I felt that it was very difficult to push her to understand the meaning of forgetting. In supervision, Dr. Stimmel helped me to see that this client was only at the mentalization level of understanding the behavior. "You have to accept that she just cannot understand that right now," said Dr. Stimmel. "Do not expect an immediate and understanding response. You can break it down into more detail, and you can ask her, 'Why aren't you interested in understanding that we both forgot the session at the same time?'" Instead of expecting the client to give me a good reflective response in that moment, I instead helped her move forward a little bit from her current state by breaking it into parts and stimulating her curiosity about the event.

High sense of self-regard and self-efficacy of the supervisor

Dr. Stimmel demonstrates high self-regard and a high sense of self-efficacy when she offers interventions and supervisory advice. At times, supervisors are taught to give supervisees brief and clear advice instead of direct feedback that can provoke feelings of discomfort. This had been one of the biggest challenges I faced in the early years of my career. At that time, even when I found that my supervisees used the wrong therapeutic interventions, it was hard for me to tell them my true thoughts directly. I was afraid to make them feel criticized, and I did not want them to see me as an unsupportive supervisor. As a result, I always undermined my own recommendations. For example, I instructed them that they should not give interpretive feedback to clients in between sessions. However, when supervisees reported that they had received messages from their clients during these intervals and were tempted into offering a therapeutic response, I would say, "It's OK for you to respond to them." I was aware of the narcissistic traits of my supervisees and sensed that my suggestions would threaten them. I wanted to protect them and avoid conflict; but, in return, the supervisees felt confused by my contradictory suggestions.

In contrast, Dr. Stimmel gave me clear and simple advice. She told me that we should follow the rule of the bare minimum when replying to our clients between sessions. She also discussed the specific replies I could give my supervisees and clients in various boundary-violating situations. All of her advice was clear, simple, consistent, and firm, which is what built the solid foundation of our supervisory relationship. On the occasions that I did not follow her advice, I was comfortable speaking with her about it and explaining how my relationship with the client made me respond differently from what she had advised.

Respect of the supervisor for the supervisee

Dr. Stimmel is very confident in her clinical judgments. However, self-confidence does not mean arrogance. She has never imposed her views on me. One of my clients once requested temporarily switching to video sessions. I discussed with the client the meaning of the change and how she was repeating her past interpersonal patterns. The client entirely agreed with me and even offered many examples that further supported my analysis. However, after our discussion, she still insisted on switching to video sessions. I experienced a deep sense of powerlessness at the time, and I was stuck. I had a conundrum. If I insisted on continuing with face-to-face sessions, I would turn into her coercive and controlling mother; but if I accepted her request for the temporary change, she would be playing the role of the controller (her mother) in our relationship. No matter what, we would still be repeating her troubled pattern.

Dr. Stimmel gave me simple advice: respect your client by insisting on face-to-face sessions while offering another option. If the client could not attend the session in person, I could suggest canceling that session. Consequently, I could insist on retaining the therapeutic setting without forcing the client to accept my request. Following this suggestion, I provided the client with two choices. Through this interaction, the client touched on a deep conflict in her life that helped her recognize that she did not passively accept the dictates of the outside world as she had thought, and then our treatment went deeper.

Dr. Stimmel's suggestion not only helped me overcome an impasse in the treatment but also embodied what it means to have respect for the client.

Dr. Stimmel not only teaches her supervisees to respect their clients; she is similarly respectful in her communications. She always gives me clear and direct suggestions, but never demands that I follow them. Some of her suggestions have conflicted with other training I have received, so I do not blindly follow her suggestions. Instead, I consider them carefully and apply them when I think it is appropriate.

For example, Dr. Stimmel and I have different policies when a patient needs to cancel or reschedule. Dr. Stimmel will offer a makeup time in the week and charges for all the sessions, even if the patient cannot attend the makeup session. My therapeutic settings are different—I allow my clients to cancel a session if they contact me at least 24 hours in advance. After clarifying this with Dr. Stimmel, I came to realize that her scheduling aims to make the treatment more consistent; she does not take this approach because the analyst, as I had initially understood, is inflexible or in a position of absolute authority. I do not use the same therapeutic frame as her, but as long as my clients and I agree on it, I will stick to it. Dr. Stimmel's respect for my own preferences has helped me maintain a high level of self-esteem and facilitates my self-reflection, which is essential for a therapist (Jacobs et al., 1995).

Strong emotional bond or attachment in the supervisory dyad

According to Jacobs (2001), Dr. Stimmel and I enacted the desire transference and countertransference that Garber (1995) said is an intrinsic element of a successful supervisory process. Attachment is the emotional bond in Bordin's (1979) theory. Bordin (1983) believed that the supervisory working alliance includes three elements: (1) supervision goals; (2) supervisory tasks; and (3) emotional bonds. I believe that emotional bonds are indispensable in forming a solid supervisory working alliance. I feel fully supported by Dr. Stimmel because of the strong emotional bond between us. No matter what problems I encounter in treatment with my clients or in supervision with my supervisees, I am able to face various difficulties more steadily, confidently, and patiently since I know that Dr. Stimmel will fully support me, correct me if I am wrong, and give me honest feedback.

For some supervisees, completing supervision hours is a necessary requirement for them to gain their postgraduate degree or graduate from certain continuing education programs. In China, where there is currently a shortage of registered supervisors, this sometimes creates problems, which I have studied by conducting interviews with Chinese supervisees in my research on supervision. Many of the supervisees I have interviewed have described feeling uncomfortable in their supervision and maybe even humiliated by their supervisors. However, they chose to stay in these unhealthy supervisory relationships in order to obtain the supervision hours they needed. Unfortunately, they were not able to develop a healthy bond with their supervisor, which, as a result, limited their ability to learn and develop their skills.

By contrast, I feel completely safe and relaxed in my supervision with Dr. Stimmel. Her great respect for me has positively influenced my supervisory relationship with her, my role as a therapist, and my role as a supervisor. In the process of interacting with her, I always feel that she treats me as a colleague. I look forward to our supervision sessions, and I am eager to discuss treatment or supervision difficulties with her. This is a marvelous experience. I completely believe in Dr. Stimmel, and I like and appreciate her very much.

Effective outcomes resulting from a good supervisory relationship

Dr. Stimmel and I have formed a mutually trusting, safe, and stable supervisory relationship, which is the foundation of effective supervision. Jacobs et al. (1995) and Jacobs (2001) explained that a positive supervisory relationship depends on the intelligence and charm of the supervisor; this in turn inspires the student to learn and entices the student to enjoy the workings of the human mind. The supervisor inspires the supervisee to reflect on the metacognitive learning process. As such, I am able to listen carefully to Dr. Stimmel's point of view without defensiveness and without feeling criticized or shamed. I can better work with the transference and countertransference in the treatments and the parallel process in the supervision. I have also learned not to criticize supervisees or threaten their self-esteem, and I give them direct and accurate feedback.

Because I trust Dr. Stimmel, even if her therapeutic and supervisory suggestions sometimes completely subvert my previous experiences, I still take them into consideration and clarify with her the reasons for making them. These are the suggestions that promote treatment and supervision, and I selectively adapt them according to my actual situation. Whenever I adopt her suggestions, I am pleasantly surprised to find that my treatment and supervision go to a depth I could not have imagined before—just like the adventures of Alice after falling down the rabbit hole.

I am not ashamed of or anxious about the blind spots or potential misunderstandings in the treatment or supervision I provide, and I am able to convey this sense of security and curiosity about the unknown in both. I have a greater understanding of my clients' traumas and defenses, and I find that I can be with them on a deeper level and appreciate their efforts in healing. My clients and I gradually accept their pains and repeated compulsions, letting the healing process happen naturally. My supervisees have also learned to reflect on their treatments with curiosity instead of shame and anxiety, which enables them to enjoy the supervision process and discover and develop their own styles. These are wonderful feelings that enable me to experience the beauty of treatment and supervision.

Having a good supervisory relationship has allowed me to work better with transference. In my practice, I am not always good at identifying the transference of the client to me, and I worry about overidentifying with them. For example, I once had a client who would change the time of our sessions at will, and I could not refuse her. At the beginning, I was not aware that I was worried that my insistence on setting a precise time would trigger her transferential anger. Through the process of supervision, I gradually came to understand my concerns, but I did not know how to deal with the client's negative transference. Subsequent supervision sessions helped me see that she regarded me as cruel, ruthless, and persecutory. I conspired with her and became wary of provoking her repressed anger. Under Dr. Stimmel's continuous supervision, I was able to detect that the client aroused my feelings of guilt, and then I could explore and understand this process with her naturally. As the treatment progressed, the client's cold and cruel world gradually became warm and inviting.

The flexibility of Dr. Stimmel's teaching has helped me learn to treat every client as a unique individual. For example, a time change for another client had a different meaning. For that client, I accepted her need to reschedule as part of my overidentification with her abuse. I was not aware of her abuse of me. She then suggested changing the time, but she forgot to consult with me again. I routinely invited her to discuss this, and she routinely gave me an objective, inviolable excuse. We only discussed it on the surface, and I did not have any other feelings about it in the process. It was as a result of Dr. Stimmel's response to it in our supervision that I felt my repressed anger rise to the surface and realized that I had been abused in the treatment. Only then was it possible to work with the client on this issue.

Having a good supervisory relationship also enables me to handle a supervisee's transference to me more calmly. The transference between the supervisee and the supervisor is not the focus of supervision, but it will affect it. Distinguishing between teaching and treating without infringing on the supervisee's boundaries is currently the biggest challenge I face in supervision. I once had a supervisee who had a very strong transference to me, and I partly identified with her projection unconsciously. I once discussed this case in a group supervision for a training program. The group supervisor pointed out the error in my supervision intervention. "Both the supervisee and her client belong to the borderline level," she said. "Allowing the supervisee to initiate the supervision at the beginning of the supervision will cause her severe regression. This client requires structured treatment, and this supervisee also needs structured supervision." The group supervisor's opinion subverted my previous understanding. I was deeply inspired by her point of view; however, her shocked facial expression and her astonished tone made me feel very bad during the teaching process. I felt very ashamed, very frustrated, and even doubted my competency to do dynamic supervision. This group supervision, like dominoes, triggered a series of self-denials. Later, I brought this supervision experience to Dr. Stimmel, and her response made me feel no shame at all. She said that the supervision was mine, and it was up to me to judge whether I could continue working with that supervisee. "You are not the only supervisor in the world, and she is not the only supervisee. You can stop the supervision if you cannot work on it," Dr. Stimmel said. What she said put me at ease. Meanwhile, she also helped me distinguish between the parallel process and transference (Quinodoz, 1994; Stimmel, 1995).

In the next session, I told the supervisee, "Some transferential enactments happened between us. It was not the parallel process and had nothing to do with the case, which has severely damaged our supervisory alliance." However, I was not her analyst, so I said, "Let's try together to readjust our supervisory relationship without analyzing it. If the transferential relationship between us no longer affects our working alliance, we will continue the supervision. If it still exists, we will terminate the supervision relationship." She agreed. She told me that at the beginning of our supervision, she felt angry at me for ignoring her. She gave me some suggestions that would enable her to use the supervision more effectively. I also gave her some suggestions for continuing to study and accepting analysis. Through the discussion, I again clarified the goals of her supervision at that stage and assisted her in continuously distinguishing between clients' emotions and those that she projected onto them. From then on, our supervision went smoother, and both of us felt very comfortable. She participated in a two-year intensive psychoanalysis training program during which we were able to gain a more focused understanding of the dynamics of her cases and also reinforce her understanding of what she had learned from her classes.

For the same supervision case, I had the experience of being supervised by two different supervisors. Both the group supervisor and Dr. Stimmel offered me their insight in very direct and clear ways, but the results were diametrically opposed. The group supervisor made me want to avoid supervision, but Dr. Stimmel enabled me to face the challenges present in the supervisory relationship. I think the essential difference was not the content of what had been suggested in the supervision, but whether the two sides of the supervisory dyad had established a strong relationship and whether I felt safe in the relationship as a supervisee. Positive and strong emotional bonds between the supervisee and the supervisor make the supervisee want to explore new situations with curiosity rather than experience frustration and shame, and subsequently want to avoid supervision when the supervisor points out their blind spots.

The above vignette also shows that a good supervisory relationship allows the supervisee to accept and digest the supervisor's feedback. Evaluation is the nucleus of clinical supervision (Bernard & Goodyear, 2019). I have always aimed to give supervisees proper evaluations and feedback, but I have not always done it well. In my first supervision training program, I learned about the "shit sandwich" approach, which suggests giving negative feedback to supervisees in between two positive points of feedback. This method may be useful for novice supervisors. When I was a novice supervisor, I really did not know how to evaluate and give feedback. But with this technique, when I wanted to point out that the supervisees were wrong, I would think about some of their merits and praise them as well. When they heard the praise and affirmation, they felt happy, thus softening the blow. But there are drawbacks to using this approach.

Firstly, whether offering praise or criticism, the supervisor will turn into an absolute authority when passing judgment on the supervisee. This undermines the goal of establishing a cooperative and equal supervisory relationship. Secondly, supervisees view the shit sandwich approach as somehow controlling or alienating, which negatively affects the genuine and trusting supervisory relationship. Thirdly, after prolonged exposure to the shit sandwich approach, supervisees become immune to praise. I found that even if I pointed out to them what they were doing well, they felt that I was just trying to comfort and encourage them, and they thought that they were actually doing a terrible job. As a result, overusing the shit sandwich approach can harm a supervisee's ability to develop their independent and confident clinical judgment. Therefore, I am always looking for a better way to give feedback.

Dr. Stimmel's supervision lets me experience effective supervisory feedback firsthand. When I make an obvious intervention error, Dr. Stimmel will point it out very clearly and inform me of other more appropriate options in that counseling scenario. She has taught me to understand my blind spots in a respectful and supportive way, and helped me distinguish between teaching and passing criticism and judgment. When she gives me corrective feedback, she repeatedly acknowledges my feelings about her assessment without rejecting or humiliating me. I can sense her care and respect for me. This consistently simple and clear attitude that is not condescending is an excellent model for me to follow. Gradually, I have become able to provide concise, clear, and firm feedback to my supervisees as well.

When I do well, Dr. Stimmel's unintentional affirmation makes me feel like I am really doing a good job. This realism not only strengthens our supervisory relationship but also makes me more independent and more confident in my counseling and judgment as a supervisor. Affirmations in the supervision are important to supervisees, as are corrective suggestions. As a supervisee, I need clear feedback. I need to know which aspects of my consultation or supervision are appropriate, which aspects are inappropriate, and how to improve. In supervision, Dr. Stimmel will never hesitate to affirm what I have done well, which makes me more confident in my treatment and supervision interventions.

Conclusion

Even though cultural and theoretical diversity could impede effective supervision, through her ingenious talents and efforts, Dr. Stimmel's approach demonstrates how to establish a good supervisory relationship and facilitate the professional growth of supervisees no matter where they come from. She is real for me even though I have only met her via video. Her realness is not only based on her unique characteristics but also on her fantastic clinical competency and high self-regard. Even though she frequently challenges and subverts my understanding, I know she respects me. Our strong emotional bond has helped me broaden my capacity for reflection and containment, both as a counselor and as a supervisor. Maintaining my curiosity and keen interest in reorganizing my existing knowledge is a wonderful feeling, and I appreciate the beauty and uncertainty of the treatment and supervision, for which I have Dr. Stimmel to thank.

Note

1 All identifying information has been disguised to protect the privacy of the client/patient. Any resemblance to actual persons, living or dead, is purely coincidental.

References

Bernard, J. M., & Goodyear, R. K. (2019). *Fundamentals of clinical supervision* (6th ed.). Pearson.

Bordin, E. S. (1979). The generalizability of the psychoanalytic concept of the working alliance. *Psychotherapy: Theory, Research & Practice*, 16(3), 252–260. doi:10.1037/h0085885.

Bordin, E. S. (1983). A working alliance-based model of supervision. *The Counseling Psychologist*, 11(1), 35–42.

Garber, M. B. (1995). *Vice versa: Bisexuality and the eroticism of everyday life* Simon & Schuster.

Gelso, C. J., & Carter, J. A. (1985). The relationship in counseling and psychotherapy: Components, consequences, and theoretical antecedents. *The Counseling Psychologist*, 13(2), 155–243. doi:10.1177/0011000085132001.

Jacobs, D. (2001). Narcissism, eroticism, and envy in the supervisory relationship. *Journal of the American Psychoanalytic Association*, 49(3), 813–829.

Jacobs, D., David, P., & Meyer, D. J. (1995). *The supervisory encounter: A guide for teachers of psychodynamic psychotherapy and psychoanalysis.* Yale University Press.

Quinodoz, J. (1994). Transference of the transference in supervisions: Transference and countertransference between the candidate-analyst and analysand when acted out in the supervision. *Journal of Clinical Psychoanalysis*, 3(4), 593–606.

Stimmel, B. (1995). Resistance to awareness of the supervisor's transference with special reference to the parallel process. *International Journal of Psycho-Analysis*, 76, 609–618.

Chapter 5

Remote supervision between Korea and New York

Overcoming cross-cultural challenges in supervision

Moosuk Lee

Introduction

I began undergoing psychoanalytic supervision with Dr. Barbara Stimmel in 2005 when I was a psychoanalytic candidate. The supervision took place once a week for over two and a half years and was conducted on the phone between Gwangju, Korea, where I resided, and New York, where Dr. Stimmel was a training analyst. I sent verbatim transcripts of sessions in English via email in advance, and then made the phone call to New York at the prearranged time. In this chapter, I am going to present the analytic process of Mrs. L, a patient with whom I worked for two and a half years, four times per week, using the analytic couch.[1] In the presentation of the case, I will integrate many notes I took, as well as notes that Dr. Stimmel emailed me after our supervision sessions. I will conclude with an in-depth description of how positively I felt that the significant cultural differences between us were handled in my supervisory relationship with Dr. Stimmel.

Analytic process of Mrs. L

Mrs. L was a 45-year-old housewife. At our first meeting, she was polite and seemed a bit nervous, but she had a bright look and spoke fairly honestly. I liked her. "What brings you here?" I asked. The reason for her visit was that her psychologist had recommended she undergo psychoanalysis. She said, "I don't know much about psychoanalysis. I just need to understand my own mind." She thought there might be certain reasons for her cold and defensive reactions to her husband—even his simply talking could upset her. She wished to understand this better and to ultimately restore the peaceful relationship they had once shared.

Her attitude toward her husband's affair was particularly unusual. When she found out that he had been living a double life with another woman for three years, she was disappointed but never pressed him on the matter; she did not get angry either. In fact, she continued carrying out all of her duties as a wife, including wiping her husband's shoes and arranging them nicely to make it easy for him to put them on when he left for work, accompanying him to the elevator, and telling him to have a nice day at work, all the while cursing him as a "crazy bastard" on the inside. At times, she would suddenly act cold toward her husband, but then she would apologize soon after. She hated how worthless, small, and insignificant she felt every time she stood before him. She said that she just wanted to know what was wrong with her.

Through analysis, we discovered that Mrs. L's behavior had an unconscious motivation. The motivation was a complex one; but, simply put, she was repeating her father and mother's internal object relationship from when she was young. This relationship was a sadomasochistic one. Her father was an adulterer and an incompetent alcoholic. He constantly beat her mother, who put up with it and let herself be victimized. Her mother would scream and run when he beat her, but she continued the tough work of feeding and taking care of her family. As a child, Mrs. L felt sorry for her mother but was unable to protect her. From her perspective as a young girl, her father was a sadist and her mother a masochist. Mrs. L's child-within kept on recreating this role play of her inner theater. She played the masochist role of her mother. This was the reason why she had not been able to express her rage to her husband. Her mother had never once rebelled against her father, opting for thorough repression of her anger instead.

Mrs. L's feelings for her husband were complex. In her unconscious, her husband was simultaneously an object of anger and a dependable guardian. Her fear of abandonment turned him into an object of strength with whom she had to ingratiate herself. She believed that it was not right to show anger even if someone was unfairly angry with her; rather, she thought it was safer to keep smiling. Mrs. L was unaware that she was angry at her husband. In fact, even I, the candidate analyst, had overlooked her repressed anger.

In discussing Mrs. L's case with Dr. Stimmel during supervision, I particularly wanted to learn how Mrs. L's repressed anger was realized. Dr. Stimmel used the notes from my ongoing sessions with Mrs. L to demonstrate her pattern of displacement. For example, the patient was angry when her husband phoned but did not express it, and then threw the phone after hanging up. Or, when she was angry at her husband, she often took it out on her son. How could anyone be unable to recognize their own emotions? I was unaware of this psychological phenomenon until I studied psychoanalysis and became aware of it through supervision. The analysis followed the story of the patient on the surface and explored the effects and fantasies that developed from within. In other words, the purpose was to help the patient think about her inner life.

Dr. Stimmel invited me to think about Mrs. L's anger and her expression of anger in her personal life as expressions of anger toward me and the psychoanalytic treatment as well. As she pointed out,

> As you get to know the patient, you will have to anticipate how she will respond as the treatment progresses. She may very likely break it off without directly expressing her anger in front of you, and especially towards you. When and if that time comes you can ask her the following, "Do you think as in your throwing the phone after speaking with your

husband rather than directly confronting him, you are doing the same here with me? Instead of throwing away a phone, you are throwing away me and your analysis?"

When I brought up the idea of anger in sessions with Mrs. L, she seemed shocked to recognize her anger: "So, I've been angry, even though I had no idea?" And although she seemed to accept this part of herself, and I was able to show her through other relationships and situations that this was a significant defense and character issue, Mrs. L was not able to easily resolve this repressed anger within. Instead, she continued to displace it to her husband's family and her second son (who resembled her husband), in particular. She used reaction formation with friends at church by repeatedly transforming anger into kindness.

Mrs. L was often late to sessions, and even missed them entirely. Doing so was an expression of her anger toward me for not recognizing her. As the idealized transference object, I was a caring holy spirit and an embracing, non-critical being. Mrs. L felt unrecognized by me, this ideal figure, with the result being that she often felt shabby, depressed, and angry after her sessions. The more ideal and holy I seemed to her, the shabbier she felt in my presence. This problem persisted from an early stage until the end of her analysis; but there was one event in particular that helped her to gain insight. I will describe the session in which this occurred below.

Mrs. L showed up late that day, as she had before. The session was set to go from 3:00 to 3:45, and 3:45 was the time she arrived. Following the contract, no psychoanalysis was performed on her that day, and she went back home. Dr. Stimmel had emphasized that I keep to the terms of the contract, stating: "The form should be respected whenever possible." I thought that Mrs. L would be angry for having to leave without anything to show for it, but, unexpectedly, she smiled and quickly blurted out: "I'm fine, doctor. I'm the one who feels sorry for making you wait, I can come back tomorrow. It's OK. Don't worry about me." She had come for a session, wasted the fee, and left empty-handed. She might have expected a psychoanalyst to be flexible with her, but she was refused. She could have been angry about it. Instead, Mrs. L was chatty and considerate of my feelings.

In planning for the next session, I knew that I had to focus on Mrs. L's actions instead of her words. Dr. Stimmel's comment in this regard will remain with me forever: "Not dealing with missed sessions is like letting a bird in the hand fly off only to land again." I remember Dr. Stimmel suggesting that when the patient is late, silent, or expresses an unexplained action, I should encourage her to think about all of this and ask, for example, "I wonder if you might have come late yesterday because you had some feelings that were difficult to express. What thoughts come to mind?" She also suggested pointing out the possibility of an acting-in by asking the question in a more open-ended way, such as, "What comes to mind about yesterday's session?" Dr. Stimmel's central point (that became an underlying concept for me) when listening in sessions is that we almost always try not to have preconceived notions, or even directions, about what "happened." This is one major aspect of cultural constraints that I will discuss below.

Similar to these enactments, Mrs. L sent me a letter that Dr. Stimmel characterized as a love letter. As with the late/missed sessions, Dr. Stimmel recommended that I not remain silent about the letter so it would not become a secret between me and the patient. She likened it to a diamond, which made me think of a *gayageum* (a Korean musical instrument). With Dr. Stimmel's guidance, I was able to use the letter as a connection between the patient and the analytic work and make sure that I, as the analyst, did not become the central character on the stage. Dr. Stimmel pointed out that, somehow, I had contributed to the patient's continuing enactment by not addressing the meaning of her action (the letter) in the session. And she suggested approaching my patient as follows: "Thank you for the letter, Mrs. L. I see that you feel grateful to me and you are taking the therapy very seriously. I hope we can try to understand the letter as having many other layers of meanings." I used Dr. Stimmel's approach in the following session, and a common action between people became a rich source of understanding of Mrs. L's inner life.

Dr. Stimmel also continued to invite me to look at the different meanings and outcomes when redirecting the focus onto the patients. For instance, she emphasized the importance of here and now transference perspectives. She said: "When the patient says something about you, do not think about it in an ordinary sense but rather in the transference context; that will assist the working through process of her experience of you as a holy spirit." It made me think about Lucifer, who was originally an angel but became a demon. I realized that the shift between idealization and devaluation needed to happen, and, for a while, that was the person I would become. Hopefully, I could finally be more ordinary—quite in between heaven and hell!

Neutrality and psychodynamic formulation

I was curious to understand the connection between neutrality and psychodynamic formulation; how much intervention is required in the analytic treatment? Sigmund Freud's (1912) paper "Recommendations to Physicians Practicing Psycho-analysis" recommends that the analyst not intervene in order to let patients associate freely. Dr. Stimmel suggested conceptualizing neutrality as reflective of the activity and passivity of the analyst. She also reminded me that neither the analyst nor the patient is alone in the room, such that there is a constant interplay between them. We might find that if the analyst is too active, the patient will become passive as a counterpoint; or if the analyst only listens and never "acts," such as interprets, the patient may become disoriented and progress will be slow. Dr. Stimmel's main concern was too much intellectualization on my part. She cautioned that I might not work "at the moment" when I intellectualize analytic processes with theoretical concepts. She emphasized the importance of "affects" that were experienced in the here and now analytic processes. When I internalized this as guidelines rather than rules, I was able to become more present and responsive to my patients.

As a candidate in psychoanalytic training, I had presuppositions based on stereotypes of the analyst. Very often I was confused as to how much I should listen and not speak without intervention; is analysis just listening and doing nothing? Dr. Stimmel was also helpful in broad conceptual thinking. She explained that psychoanalytic thinking is based on thinking together as the analyst helps the patient let go of as many resistances to free association as possible. She encouraged me not to try to find and say the perfect thing; equally imperative is not to expect the perfect answer from the patient. Instead, I should give both the patient and myself room to learn together. She modeled this through her supervision style.

Back to Mrs. L, I said to her: "You showed up for your session yesterday just as the hour was ending, you weren't able to meet with me and you went back home. What do you feel or think about that?" She responded that she was sorry for wasting my valuable time the day before. She continued in a distressed tone: "Why do I always do such stupid things? I was worried that you might say that you didn't want to see a person like me anymore." What emerged was that she had actually been afraid of being abandoned by me for over two years during our sessions. To her, I said:

> Although you came late to the session, you did show up and you paid the fee. So it seems that you are the one who lost out, not me, because you paid without receiving any psychoanalysis. But instead, you are concerning yourself with my feelings and trying to comfort me. What could be the reason for that; does anything come to mind?

She replied, "Maybe I've mentioned this before, but there's one thing that comes to my mind at the moment." And then she shared the following memory from her childhood.

When Mrs. L was ten years old, her mother sent her to live with her maternal grandparents due to her father's pulmonary tuberculosis. She lived there for one year while her older brother and younger sister stayed with her parents. It was unfair. She showed symptoms of childhood neurosis through separation anxiety at that time, such as stealing and enuresis. But they disappeared just after her reunion with her parents. When at her maternal grandparents' house she would pretend to be cheerful when her mother showed up, making comments such as "Mom, I like being at your parents' house" and "My aunts were nice enough to buy me some clothes. Don't worry about me." She would do everything she could to reassure her mother out of fear of being left there indefinitely if she offended her. Mrs. L realized that her habit of considering the feelings of others and trying to make them feel good stemmed from the events that happened while at her grandparents' house; to prevent complete abandonment by her mother, she pretended to be comfortable—even happy.

That memory, profound as it was, did not include any recognition of the rage she felt at her mother's rejection. When she arranged to be unable to have an analytic session with me the previous day, she was enacting all aspects of the memory, with the rage being directed at herself for having done such a "stupid thing." I was forced into the role of her abandoning mother. In addition, we could learn more of her need to idealize me as a way to control her pain and anger toward me in the transference. And we could quickly apply this to the behavior in her marriage. She knew that her husband was cheating on her (much as her mother did by keeping her brother and sister at home), and yet she had to ingratiate herself with him due to her fear of abandonment. The only way to manage the anger was to repress it and then displace it to others. And, as she did with me, she used idealization to defend herself and him against the anger that terrified her. We could also identify her "kindness" as a different defense against her anger, and this reversal also included changing rage and hatred to idealization and glorification.

It was in this context that Dr. Stimmel was invaluable in helping me understand the nature and use of the transference. I came to see that by continually going back and forth between Mrs. L's relationships with others and her relationship with me, we were able to work through much of Mrs. L's repressed rage and fear of loss. But then Dr. Stimmel asked me to turn the lens onto myself. She suggested that in the face of Mrs. L's unceasing aggression, I was employing my own form of avoidance. We began to work on my discomfort in looking at the aggression (yet another cultural divide that will be discussed below). Although the patient was avoiding her own aggression by dreaming of attacking her brother, missing sessions, or not calling me to let me know that she would be late for the sessions, I experienced a different form of attack. Mrs. L's provocative behaviors were their own brand of reaction formation, which allowed me to be "better" than her; and, understandably, they also fueled her own neurotic need to idealize the very person who was hurting her the most.

For example, I was bothered by the fact that Mrs. L was linking the wishes of her father or husband to die with the actual act of killing; these frightening fantasies led to immense guilt. It was difficult for me to do much with these thoughts, even as I was sure I was one of her intended victims. It seemed easier for me to keep all this at arm's length and talk about it in the abstract. My fear, rage, and sense of failure were dictating this passivity. With Dr. Stimmel's help, I was able to deal directly with Mrs. L's wishes and work out my own transference toward her along the way.

Another aspect of my work with Dr. Stimmel had to do with thinking about how the mind works for and against the patient. For example, I wondered if lust in the heart constitutes adultery. Can thought alone be sinful? Dr. Stimmel helped me accept that as long as the patient does not act on her wishes, they remain just that—wishes. A very important precept she helped me incorporate is the basic conviction that human beings can and do think forbidden thoughts. I was able to dispel my own belief that thinking can be a sin; otherwise, I would have continued to face significant limitations in my work as a psychoanalyst when treating my patients, since all of them have terrifying negative wishes.

Termination

We were now at the end of the analysis. I had helped Mrs. L understand some of her inner conflicts that made her unhappy. Through transference interpretation, she was able to experience the conflict in a real way. However, she could not/would not relinquish her desire for an object of infinite love and care. This resistance manifested in arriving late and missing sessions, and, although we repeatedly dealt with these issues, her resistance was persistent. Then one day, she said that she wanted to quit the analysis, citing cost as the reason.

She had been considering filing for divorce, and had been secretly putting money aside to prepare for that eventuality. However, any thoughts of divorce disappeared during the psychoanalysis. She told her husband about the secret funds, and in so doing, she lost her source of money to pay for the psychoanalysis. Not only had she been keeping the money a secret, she had also been keeping the sessions a secret from her husband. It became clear to both of us that there were multiple reasons for her to tell her husband about the money and the analysis—among them was the necessity to stop treatment. This wish to stop analysis became strongest in the context of dealing with her repressed aggression. It seemed obvious that she was unwilling to move further along in giving up this complicated and neurotic wish fulfillment.

When I brought this up in supervision, Dr. Stimmel validated my thought that the patient's reasons for talking about termination paradoxically included her fear of ending her relationship with me. She was sure I would not allow her to come back once I recognized that I was central among her planned victims of love and death. Dr. Stimmel suggested that I ask her: "What comes to mind about the words 'ending it?'"

When beginning the analysis, Mrs. L had two goals. One was to understand her own feelings, and the other was to restore a peaceful relationship with her husband. These goals were partially attained. Her relationship with her husband had improved, and she no longer took out her anger on her family. She said that she was happy. I respected her financial difficulty even though there were a lot of tasks remaining to be dealt with analytically. I agreed with her decision to quit analysis and said, "I appreciate the work we did together. If you want to see me, don't hesitate to call me. My door is always open for you."

Supervisee's transference

I had an unusual experience when my supervision with Dr. Stimmel had been going on for about a year. Mrs. L was often absent or late to sessions, and that had been analyzed as transference resistance. For example, the patient had seen me as an ideal object and wanted to be recognized by me. The patient perceived me as a critical teacher and played the part of a good student in order to avoid punishment. She was ashamed and nervous in front of me, believing herself to be an incompetent and boring patient. Compared to her, I was a skilled and experienced analyst. This transference resistance had been dealt with repeatedly throughout my supervision with Dr. Stimmel. However, the patient continued to arrive late or miss sessions.

Then one day, the supervision time started to feel like a burden to me. I felt like an incompetent supervisee. It seemed like this competent and internationally well-recognized supervisor was disappointed in me and thought of me as having no hope for improvement. Just thinking about supervision time made me nervous and depressed. What particularly bothered me was the sound of Dr. Stimmel sighing, which I could hear coming through the phone. It sounded like a sigh of disappointment, a sigh that said: "You're not making any progress because you don't know how to do any better." To me, she was infinitely superior, and, compared to her, I was small and inferior. About two months after this, I discussed my painful feelings with my other supervisor. He empathized with me and said: "Every supervisor has their own supervision style. You might have interpreted your supervisor's type as blame." That comforted me, but the tension continued.

Finally, I told Dr. Stimmel about my emotional state. We discussed the matter in depth, and she was surprised to hear this unexpected story of mine. She was very concerned that I had been feeling this way, especially for such a long period. She was particularly interested in the sighing I described. We talked about the unavoidable comparison I had made between myself and the patient, and in turn between Dr. Stimmel and myself. I was three people with Dr. Stimmel: the patient, the analyst, and the supervisee. During this discussion, I saw clearly how the disappointing self I had described to Dr. Stimmel was exactly how the patient had described herself with me. The ideal figure in my case was my supervisor. In other words, the transference that had emerged between the patient and me was reproduced between me (the supervisee) and Dr. Stimmel (the supervisor). We spent some time discussing the parallel process, and that allowed Dr. Stimmel to consider how she had played her part in this duplication of the primary therapeutic relationship. Dr. Stimmel reassured me that she was neither disappointed nor disapproving of my work. She did not experience the sighing, and wondered if indeed it had occurred, even while accepting that perhaps it had because she too has an unconscious! I believe Dr. Stimmel's sighing was a figment of my imagination.

After that discussion, I received supervision for another year and a half but never heard another sigh. I became comfortable again, and what I was most thankful for was the chance to have an earnest experience and empathize with the psychological reality of my patient. Throughout our supervisions, Dr. Stimmel always demonstrated that a good teacher is also open to her students' ideas. This concept was also true in psychoanalytic thinking, which is based on being comfortable and thinking together. It helped me a great deal when listening to Mrs. L, and she came up with thoughts different to mine. After all, there is no one answer. At times, I was worried that my answers were not good enough or that I would be perceived as not smart. Dr. Stimmel's voice would then be in my mind: "Help the patient help you; accept her different perspective, and together you will grow."

Cultural differences

Dr. Stimmel always showed an interest in the personal meaning and impact of cultural tradition on the individual and the treatment. She would highlight that we understand our patients through our own and shared cultural experiences. To that end, she tried to learn as much as she could about the differences between our two cultures in order for her to understand both me and Mrs. L better. She said that would help the treatment come alive during the supervisory sessions.

For example, Mrs. L had two sons, but she could not remember the age of the older one. However, she knew he was born in the year of the rat. As a Korean, Mrs. L's use of the term "the year of the rat" was for me a normal way of stating someone's age. However, for Dr. Stimmel, it was a new concept that required further explanation and maybe new meaning in the inner life of the patient. Koreans use 12 animals that each symbolize one year in the Chinese zodiac; thus, every 12 years, the same animal returns. These years and animals carry a special meaning when it comes to a person's fate. Those born in the year of the rat, for example, are said to have plenty to eat and end up rich if they are born at night. Meanwhile, those born in this year during the daytime are said to end up unhappy with nothing to eat. Mrs. L's eldest son was born in this year, and I learned that Mrs. L was too—both were born during the day and thus fated to a life of misery. Within the supervision, I began to consider how Mrs. L had a particular love for her eldest son while she hated her second son, who resembled her husband. She used this cultural tradition to align herself with her eldest son.

Korean culture and authority

During the supervision, Dr. Stimmel noted that the patient's transference of idealization may have been related to aspects of Korean culture. She was right. Korean culture has at its center the tradition of holding the utmost respect for authority. We are taught not even to step on a teacher's shadow out of respect. We must use honorific language when speaking with our elders, regardless of the age difference—one year is the same as several. For example, students salute their elders when they see them, even when they are only a single grade above them. At the dinner table, Koreans are not permitted to start eating until the father picks up his spoon. It is no surprise then that this would all manifest in our clinical work.

I had not seen this as a separate set of issues and fantasies that could actually be worked through since it is so embedded in my relationships as well. Ironically, the fact that Dr. Stimmel was unused to this cultural difference allowed her to help me see that it was also a defense, a resistance, and an essential part of the transference/countertransference relationship. It was embedded in the reasons why the patient idealized me and saw me as an authority figure. But, equally important, I saw myself as an authority figure. I was the professor, the doctor, the elder, and the man—I stepped into this role automatically. This arrangement between two people was so familiar to me that it interfered with my recognizing how this was affecting our work. It took much work on my part to begin to unravel these threads.

Another aspect of the impact of culture on the analytic work was in relation to how aggression is managed in Korea. As with lines of authority, there are rigid lines around strong expressions of emotion so that Mrs. L's defenses, idealization, and reaction formation, in particular, were almost automatic across our society. The advantage of having a supervisor from another culture outweighed the complications. Dr. Stimmel was able to wonder with me about things that I took for granted. And, most importantly, we came to understand how these differences were having an impact on our supervision. I am a Korean supervisee and must respect the authority of Dr. Stimmel. And, as we saw above, this led to a complex reaction of my own to the experience of supervision itself. Nevertheless, as I mentioned earlier, Dr. Stimmel has always demonstrated that a good teacher is also open to a student's new ideas. This was so novel to me that I actually did not take it seriously, at least not at first.

Providing analysis in the Korean language and receiving supervision in English and over the phone is challenging. As a supervisee, I had to put in a lot of effort before each session. I would send Dr. Stimmel notes, in English, on my sessions with Mrs. L. I wanted Dr. Stimmel to have the materials in our supervisory meetings so she would not spend too much time trying to understand me. Dr. Stimmel encouraged me to ask questions and to express my opinions. When she had trouble following my halting English, I appreciated how she said one "pardon?" after another. Dr. Stimmel never hesitated to ask me clarifying questions. She was genuinely interested in my work with Mrs. L and always asked me to provide more details. I was challenged by her because I did not always have the answers.

Dr. Stimmel was kind enough to understand how our cultural differences could impact my learning and treatment of patients. As a result, she would type out emails with additional explanations for the parts of the supervision that I did not understand over the phone; this was extremely helpful. I was able to translate the notes into Korean on my own time and later use them with many other patients.

Appreciation for Dr. Barbara Stimmel

I was very fortunate to have Dr. Stimmel as a supervisor. She taught me the essential knowledge that I needed as a junior analyst. Fifteen years later, I am a training analyst, and her advice still comes to mind when I am analyzing patients or doing supervision. She gives me direction from within.

Although I felt nervous when starting my supervision with Dr. Stimmel, in the end, I felt the joy of enlightenment through shining a light on the once ambiguous inner world of the patient. Dr. Stimmel jokingly called this experience "the elephant in the room." Despite the time difference between Gwangju and New York resulting in some very early supervision times, I do not remember Dr. Stimmel ever missing a session. I also introduced her to analytic candidate analysts here in Korea. I think of Dr. Stimmel as a true treasure in the International Psychoanalytic Association, and would like to take this opportunity to express my thanks.

Thank you so much, Dr. Stimmel!

Note

1 All identifying information has been disguised to protect the privacy of the client/patient. Any resemblance to actual persons, living or dead, is purely coincidental.

Reference

Freud, S. (1912). Recommendations to physicians practicing psycho-analysis. *The standard edition of the complete psychological works of Sigmund Freud. Volume XII (1911–1913): The case of Schreber.* Papers on Technique and Other Works, 12. Hogarth.

Chapter 6

Embarking on the journey of psychoanalytic supervision

The supervisor as the fixer

Camille Maruccia-Lee

Introduction

My relationship with Barbara Stimmel began when I was a candidate at the New York Freudian Society—now called the Contemporary Freudian Society (CFS)—in 1989. She was the instructor for the early Freud course, which started at 8 o'clock at night. Like most of my fellow candidates, I was blurry-eyed and weary after a full day of work. While we were discussing Freud's *Three Essays*, I picked up a glass pitcher to pour myself some water and lost my grip; the pitcher fell to the floor, sending shattered glass all over. Everyone turned around to look at me, and I was mortified by my clumsy mistake—this was not the introduction to the class I had been hoping for.

The following week, when we entered the room, I looked over at the table to see the pitcher in one piece. Barbara explained that she and her husband had put it together with glue over the weekend. I was touched by her sensitivity. Despite her tough exterior, she was also kind-hearted. She loved what she was doing, was passionate about the work, and had a great deal of energy even at that hour. I wanted to be just like her.

In my mind, Barbara came to be known as "the fixer." She could fix pitchers as well as cases. Cases came to us broken, and yet she always had some idea of how to put them back together through psychoanalysis—not by magic. Psychoanalysis seems like a painful endeavor at times; it requires patience, time, and discipline to be an analyst. In that class, I had no idea what I was undertaking or the years it would take for me to finish my training. Barbara once described the case of a woman who had been in psychoanalysis for many years who finally came to accept herself after leaving the analytic napkin on the sofa when she left the session. Before that, she would always take it with her—but she had finally stopped thinking of herself as dirty, smelly, or foul. I was in awe. From this brief description of a long analysis, I began to get an idea of how Barbara worked, and I was intrigued.

Years after the mishap with the glass pitcher, I went to see Barbara about a control case that was not going very well—a case I needed in order to graduate from the New York Freudian Society institute.[1] She listened as I told her about a man who had been in psychoanalysis four times a week; and then she told me some things that I did not want to hear, namely, that the man was too fragile and disorganized to be in psychoanalysis. Although he appeared to be well put together, he was somehow unfit for this kind of treatment. Deep down, I knew that she was right. After digesting the news and mourning the loss of a control case to present, we started talking about another case—that of a woman who was just starting analysis with me and who would be both dynamically and interpersonally complicated. Barbara said that she would supervise the case.

I considered the patient a countertransference minefield. Although small and slight in build, the patient's words packed a punch and were mostly aimed to inflict maximum damage. In turn, I feared exposing my innermost feelings (mostly anger, negativity, and some envy) in supervision. I was not comfortable thinking or talking about my aggression toward the patient, so I did the opposite. I bent over backward to appease the patient, which was somewhat a reaction formation, and instead of being grateful, the patient demanded more from me.

Barbara was not very happy with my appeasing act toward the patient. When I made up a session for the patient without exploring its meaning, she questioned me about it in a non-confrontational sort of way. I was a little frightened of Barbara as well, as aspects of her reminded me of my mother, but I wanted to learn from her, so I tried to explore its meaning in the next session with the patient. At first, the patient shrugged off my inquiry, but I persisted, and it led to an important breakthrough. The patient saw my making up of missed sessions as a way of demonstrating my love and affection for her, which was an act she fantasized meant that she was a favored child-patient. She also got me to do something for her (make up the session) that she really did not need but desperately wanted.

In supervision, I continued to fear my feelings, which Barbara sensed. As I was relatively new to the profession, I did not feel comfortable talking about my feelings out loud. I had grown up in a family where vulnerability and exposure were not encouraged. Barbara helped me relax, but not too much! By providing a holding environment, as Levenson (1982) writes about in his paper on supervisory relationships, she allowed me the space to explore some of my not-so-nice feelings. She dug deeper into some of the roots of my reactions, finding the ghosts of significant people from my own past as well as in my own analysis. I realized that some of my countertransference problems derived from a difficult relationship I had with a younger sister, who could terrorize me in a similar way to the patient. The sessions reminded me of how I suffered in silence after experiencing similar attacks in my own childhood.

Part of my worry was that some of the aggression I felt toward the patient's provocations would seep out of me, which ultimately did happen on one rare occasion during the patient's second pregnancy, when I forgot to mention that I had painted my office before her arrival. This reminded me of the time I gave my sister a peanut butter sandwich and told her it was something else (she hated peanuts) after she had gotten me in trouble with our mother.

Although always considerate and mindful of privacy concerns, I felt safe and supported in Barbara's office. I was always struck by the fact that her office seemed safe behind huge gates that led to a labyrinth of doors, mirrors, and springtime flowers off Park Avenue. Like Barbara, her office was a maze—kind of like a puzzle. Despite her Freudian-style orientation, she was open and chatty as a supervisor, offering tea, biscuits, and articles to read.

From the start, Barbara was clear with me about the patient: it was going to be rough. She was filled with envy, anger, and rage, and I became the target of her projected discontent with herself. Unhappily married, when the patient was pregnant with her first child, it stirred up fantasies of wanting to hurt the invader that had taken over her fit body. She lorded over me how easily pregnancy had come to her; but all she could rely upon was her body—it could make babies, but she did not know what else she could produce.

I learned from Barbara that the patient was deeply narcissistic; she enacted a transference alternating between a grandiose, entitled, and superior self and a depreciated, devalued, inferior object. The inferior self was mostly projected onto me. The devalued object I had become represented the patient's dissociated, regressed, and projected infantile self. My comments were often discarded, ignored, examined, and then tossed aside. She compared me to her male psychiatrist who was, according to her, of superior intelligence and knowledge than I was as a lowly woman with an inferior degree. When she was not putting me down for my age, professional choices, or looks, she simply ignored me. She did not accept being a woman herself or my being a woman. We were second-class citizens.

Nonetheless, the patient had a terrible time accepting her dependence on me. When I brought up our relationship, she talked over my comments and launched into a discussion of her problems at work with a difficult boss. A part of me was happy to leave it as it was, so as not to open Pandora's box. Barbara would hear this in the process recording, stop me, and point out that I had missed an opportunity to open up the patient's feelings about the treatment after she made that thinly veiled comment about her demanding boss that was really in reference to me. The patient felt that all I did was expect more and more work from her!

When the patient learned that I lived in Greenwich Village, my stock with her soared. She saw me as a person with an ideal life. However, this view was short-lived as the patient resumed her attacks after my long August vacation. I had disappointed her, let her down, and pulled the rug out from underneath her. My stock plummeted.

At some point, Barbara explained to me what was behind the patient's attacks. Unbeknownst to the patient, Barbara said that her attacks involved a great deal of envy toward me. The patient could not look at her deeper feelings; she found me helpful, and since it came across that I was mostly content with myself (something the patient was sorely lacking), she was envious. The patient had a history of mistreating and belittling service workers in restaurants and taxi cabs, but still, her attacks made me wince.

Complicating matters was the fact that I needed this patient in order to continue working toward my institute requirement, which made me anxious and somewhat inhibited. What if she left? Sometimes she threatened to find another therapist, like shifting her loyalty from her mother to her father. I would certainly feel badly then. I was also worried about disappointing the patient, my supervisor, and myself. Control cases were hard to come by, and since I worried about losing the patient, I held back my interpretations and protocols. Money and undercharging were also issues that Barbara encouraged me to look at. Over time, I came to realize that the patient needed me and the treatment and could not stop.

In the second year of supervision, Barbara and I turned to the patient's history, since that was important in understanding the patient's problems. The patient had a deeply narcissistic, but also loving, mother who could not get out of bed due to a debilitating depression that the patient thought was the result of a brain abnormality that ran in the family. The patient and her mother had been inseparable early on in her life; she had an intensely ambivalent and symbiotic relationship with her mother and a seductive but distant and sometimes violent relationship with her father. She was the youngest child of three and the only girl, who her father described as a "bonus." As the patient reached college age, her mother threatened to kick her out.

As a remembering, she sought this symbiotic union with me through what became a nightly practice of calling my office at 2 am, hoping that I would be available to speak with and comfort her. This was a practice the patient regularly engaged in with her closest friends as well, although some were more sympathetic and accommodating than others. We talked about this act. She hated her dependence on me, but when we were apart, it felt like she had cut off an arm or leg—she was less of a person. She sought to eliminate this feeling of loss through the ritual of calling me late at night. Why was I not available to her at all hours like a mother is to a child? With boundaries blurred, she wished for a return to that early symbiotic bliss.

In the middle of this difficult period exploring her intensely ambivalent dislike of/love for me, the patient left my Greenwich Village office near Sixth Avenue on a bright blue and sunny Thursday morning in September and saw a plane hit the World Trade Center. I was not far behind her when I left my office to head for supervision with Barbara. Somehow, I managed to reach Barbara by using a payphone (no cell phones!) and said that I had seen a plane hit the building and watched the first tower start to crumble. Barbara's voice started to crack; she sounded deeply troubled as I imagined her sitting on the edge of her seat. I overheard someone say they were bombing Washington and I scurried home.

After this incident, the patient unraveled. She had just had her first child, and, between having postpartum depression and living through 9/11, she was sinking fast into a delusional haze. She began to have fantasies of anthrax in sandboxes, and I worried for her young daughter. She went for a psychiatric evaluation. In some ways, the 9/11 attacks initiated a deep state of mourning for her; every time she went up Sixth Avenue and looked over at the empty skyline, she became despondent. I felt a bit wobbly, too. Barbara was steady and supportive, and insisted that the patient's references to 9/11 harkened back to earlier remembrances, traumas, and conflicts. She encouraged me to look at the patient's associations, daydreams, and dream life. I had not thought of it that way. The patient presented a dream about the towers falling. Like the twin towers, this dream had a double meaning: she saw us as twins who could do everything together and always be together, but that union would eventually have to come to an end. Her wish from long ago as a child was never to leave her mother's side. But, because of 9/11, she feared our union would implode—that one day, she would come to the office and find that I had left without a word of warning.

This was a very useful period of time in our work together. The patient had started to understand that the roots of her unhappiness were internal and not external. She did not like herself very much. She had never liked how her face looked, and she walked into a steel plate after leaving my office one day, breaking her nose. She blamed me. But her focus shifted after the broken nose. Her attacks lessened, and she turned to the roots of her unhappiness instead. She decided to leave her husband, which was a separation that had been many years in the making. She reunited with a childhood love. I made some decisions, too. I decided to present the case when the patient had shown some signs of improvement. Oddly, I found myself calling Barbara's office phone in the middle of the night to leave a message, telling her that the meeting with the final case committee had gone well.

After I graduated from the institute, I met with Barbara for our weekly meeting, and she turned to me and said that I was ready to stop seeing her. She offered to continue to supervise me as a colleague from time to time or as needed. I was shocked by her confidence in me, and I may have looked a bit worried. She assured me that I was ready to begin seeing the patient alone, without her guidance. For a couple of months after that, I felt a little lost. When our usual appointment time came around each week, I found that I missed our meetings. But I had the impression that Barbara believed that analysis and supervision should not go on forever, that people need to "graduate" and learn to fly solo.

For a long time after that, her advice stayed with me—particularly two of her insights. One dealt with the handling of the transference. She advised me always to "anchor" (her word) the treatment in the transference and work from there. I think she said that because many of my interventions aimed away from the transference.

Her second piece of advice was more complicated. She said that whenever someone entered my office as a new patient, I should think about my feelings toward them. It made sense. At the annual American Psychoanalytic Association conference, I find myself saying the same to colleagues. When I recently heard Barbara speak of a case, I thought I would have done the exact same thing.

Despite the abrupt ending of our supervision, Barbara continued to support me over the years. When I was at a loss for words or felt in over my head during a patient's attack, I would think of something that Barbara had said.

In her own way, in those moments, she would remind me to anchor the patient in the transference or think about how the patient started the session, and I would then feel a sense of relief. I am pleased at how much I have retained from this experience and will pass it onto others.

Note

1 All identifying information has been disguised to protect the privacy of the client/patient. Any resemblance to actual persons, living or dead, is purely coincidental.

Reference

Levenson, E. A. (1982). Follow the fox: An inquiry into the vicissitudes of psychoanalytic supervision. *Contemporary Psychoanalysis*, 18(1), 1–15.

Chapter 7

Psychodynamic supervision in the nonprofit sector

Ally Barlow

Introduction

As a social worker of nearly eight years, with many additional years of social work-adjacent experience, I am well acquainted with the role and importance of the clinical supervisor in a social work setting. I have had both truly powerful and truly underwhelming experiences with clinical supervision that have further clarified not only what I need personally from the relationship but also what qualities I expect any clinical supervisor to embody in order to engage in best practices and fully support the social worker or clinician whom they are charged to supervise.

In this chapter, I will discuss the organization within which I work as well as the specific and differentiated clinical supervision needs of clinicians in roles such as mine. I will then focus the majority of my writing on one clinical supervisor in particular, Dr. Barbara Stimmel, from whom I have received a unique type of supervision that has been deeply valuable to my practice and without whom my work would be bereft of a very significant and multifaceted type of clinical support. As I write, I will further articulate the uniqueness of my relationship with Barbara in relation to the broader context of clinical supervision for social workers.

This chapter will highlight the importance of clinical supervision even beyond obtaining clinical social work licensure. I note this specifically because it is common practice in the organizations and agencies in which I have worked to offer clinical supervision to licensed master social workers (a licensure that requires receiving weekly clinical supervision in order to practice psychotherapy). After three years of supervised practice, and once the licensed clinical social worker (LCSW) license has been obtained (a clinical licensure granting the holder the ability to independently practice psychotherapy, among other privileges), many of these organizations and agencies expect that the social worker no longer needs clinical support. This is an unfortunate, and often money-driven, narrative within the field. Clinical supervision should not exist solely to comply with state regulation, but to support and nurture the lifelong journey of a clinician as they engage in this difficult, and at times quite internal, work.

It is my hope that throughout the following chapter, the necessity of clinical supervision, as demonstrated through one very special relationship, will become increasingly clear.

Current work and role

Currently, I work in a nonprofit, community-based organization in the South Bronx in New York City that offers year-round programming to families and children. It uses the "community-to-career" approach, which prioritizes building long-term relationships and supporting members of the community's access to the academic, social, and mental health tools they need in order to advance their educational and professional goals. In addition to hosting a number of after-school programs for children of all ages (from birth through high school and well into their college and/or early professional years), the organization includes a family support and mental health team, called the Family Project, that provides holistic case management and short-term mental health counseling and therapy to individuals engaged in the programming who express an interest.

As an LCSW, I work as the Family Project's director, and occupy a number of roles within the organization. The team I supervise includes two case managers and a social work intern. My role includes maintaining a small caseload of families; meeting with clients of various ages (some children, some parents, and/or other caregivers) for weekly therapy; maintaining relationships with outside referral agencies in order to best facilitate warm handoffs for longer-term mental health care for our clients; and managing a number of projects that bring resources and materials directly to the children and families of the Hunts Point neighborhood, such as ongoing coat drives, diapers for a local family shelter, holiday gifts for children in December, and more.

My supervisees maintain larger case management caseloads. Their work includes building service plans with families, accompanying them to appointments, and advocating for public benefits and supports as needed in domains such as medical, housing, mental health, and more.

Working with Barbara

Barbara offered her services to me and to my organization on a number of fronts. In this chapter, I am going to primarily focus on the more formal relationship we engaged in, beginning in April 2019; but I would also like to note the generous informal offerings that Barbara provided even well before then. What is deeply special and unique about Barbara's work with the organization is that she has offered holistic and multi-pronged support that is quite different from the type of supervision that is rooted in classical Freudian analysis, which is her primary modality. This willingness speaks not only to her capacity and skill as a supervisor but also to her remarkable flexibility and readiness to step outside of the cultural norm of clinical supervision in order to most effectively support those with whom she comes into professional contact. The special quality of care that Barbara offers has been abundantly evident in each of my interactions with her over the years.

My first communication with Barbara took place in June 2016, when I was a year and a half into my work with the organization. A family on my caseload, which included a teenage daughter with a history of trauma and intermittent acute therapeutic need, brought Barbara to my attention as I learned that the daughter had been a pro bono client of hers in the past.[1] The young client had over the previous week expressed a desire to reconnect with Barbara because she felt that she could use clinical support for issues arising in her life. Knowing the young woman and the family quite well, I was immediately impressed with her ability to name a mental health need and request support. That she requested Barbara specifically spoke volumes; clearly, Barbara had made a significant impression on her. Furthermore, Barbara had offered this young woman care and support she certainly would not have had the resources to access otherwise. This was an apt introduction to Barbara and her work. Although Barbara and I would not engage more formally for several years, the level of her commitment and care even at that time was abundantly clear to me.

In the fall of 2018, I was advised to reach out to Barbara for a second time when working with a family with a teenage son who was demonstrating symptoms of trauma following the violent death of his classmate and close friend, who had been the victim of random and non-targeted gun violence. Barbara immediately made time to discuss the matter and support me in thinking through referral options, including offering a number of free sessions with her if that would be the most efficacious option. Barbara would, over the years, continue to offer her services in this manner—simultaneously untraditional and deeply generous—thereby granting me both an audience and conversation through this sort of intermittent clinical supervision consulting.

In April 2019, we began to engage in more structured monthly meetings, or "mini trainings," that would comprise not only the most consistent work we did together but also the deepest clinical supervision and support that Barbara would offer me over the course of our relationship. About one month prior, Barbara and I began discussing how she could offer clinical support to and build capacity within the Family Project, such as through monthly visits. After entertaining a number of ideas, we agreed to pilot a monthly meeting between Barbara, two case managers, a social work intern, and me. During these meetings, Barbara would conversationally and interactively present on a topic of our choosing, including topics such as psychoanalytic theory, the application of psychodynamic practice in an organizational setting, boundary maintenance in non-traditional settings, supporting couples and families, and many more. Barbara granted the group free rein to identify the topic, demonstrating her egolessness and very clear desire to support us in the ways that worked best for us, rather than in the ways that were most comfortable and easy for her.

Over time, we also came to integrate case conferencing into those sessions, allowing for role play and discussions of concrete matters and families with whom we worked in the Family Project. In the following four sections, I will expound on a few key elements of the work that demonstrate the quality and flexibility of Barbara's supervision.

Levels of supervision

One unexpected and fascinating element of Barbara's work with the Family Project team and her intermittent supervision of me, as requested, has been the supervisory layering of the experience. Given that Barbara has offered me a variety of forms of supervision while I supervise a number of other staff, I have been able to integrate the valuable knowledge I have received through my conversations with her into my supervisory work with my staff in real time. Furthermore, at points in the work and during the mini training sessions, I have had the opportunity and privilege to observe Barbara offering feedback and supervision to my teammates, whom I directly supervise otherwise. In this way, Barbara has modeled supervisory best practices to me both directly (through our one-on-one moments of supervision) and indirectly (through my observations of her supervision of others). This has had a significant impact on my efficacy as a supervisor, which I will describe in further detail later in the chapter.

One way in which this layered supervision experience manifested was by watching Barbara specifically advise one of my supervisees on the exploratory questions she could ask with regard to her work in a conflictual mother/daughter dyad. While I had already practiced within my work techniques similar to those that Barbara was recommending, observing Barbara make a similar suggestion to one of my supervisees both further cemented my access to that technique within my practice and demonstrated to me how best to encourage my own supervisees to utilize it. Despite often being both supervisees and supervisors, engaging in this type of observation is not an opportunity that many clinicians have over the course of their work, and it represents one of the unique elements of my work with Barbara.

Power dynamics in the supervisory relationship

Early in our work together, I became acutely aware of the power dynamics at play given that I had originally been introduced to Barbara by a board member of the organization. Within a nonprofit structure, the board is essentially the boss's boss—the arbiters of any concern with regard to the executive leadership of the organization. As such, there tends to be a high level of care taken in interactions with board members. When I was introduced to the notion of working monthly with Barbara, as per a board member's suggestion, I certainly had the option and power to say no, but I was careful to consider the implications of such a decision. Given my awareness of the weight and impact of power and relationships, it is perhaps unsurprising that I expressed a fair amount of deference to Barbara and a willingness to go along with what she thought was best. Barbara quickly disavowed me of my ingratiating attitude and quickly made it apparent that she expected me to be honest, direct, and clear in my desires and expectations for our work together, and, perhaps most importantly, challenge her as necessary. Barbara pointed to her explicit and consistent goal: to support the organization by way of our sessions together; and, as such, she expected me to clearly name the sort of supervisory and clinical support that would be best utilized given the specifics of the work and the subjectivities of the staff.

Barbara immediately paved the way for a relationship built on honesty and mutual motivation, inspired by the goal of bettering the staff and the families and children whom we serve. I note this particular quality of the work to highlight the impact of Barbara's framing and utilization of power differentials—she dismissed my deference to her power and instead expected me to be direct and truthful with her. This allowed us to dive deeply into the work in ways that were most effective and most beneficial for the clients.

Navigating differing theoretical orientations

Another special and important quality that Barbara has brought to our work is a flexibility and willingness to supervise outside of her specific professional orientation as a psychoanalytic practitioner. Within psychoanalysis, treatment boundaries are quite clear and explicit, and breaking them would quickly compromise the work. One example that stands out and demonstrates this quality occurred early on in our work together. Barbara had encouraged me to share with her a current ethical or clinical dilemma with which I was grappling. I described a situation in which I had been working with a young woman over the course of five years. When I had first met with this client, she was a 16-year-old who had previously had a stellar academic record but whose grades had recently begun slipping. One week prior to my meeting her, she had—for the first time in what would eventually amount to several times—been hospitalized after reporting persistent suicidal ideation and a strong desire to die. Over the course of the next three years, this young woman and I spent a great deal of time together. Although I was not her therapist, her family had been receiving case management services from my team for over five years already, and, as such, the young woman and her mother felt comfortable with my coordinating her care and maintaining communication with her other service providers. I also came to understand that the young woman had a history of severe childhood trauma, and at the age of 16, she was only just starting to remember, explore, and accept some of her most horrific traumatic experiences.

There were points over the course of our relationship that I offered deeply therapeutic support to this young woman during periods when she was in between consistent clinical mental health care, as she adjusted to a step-down following a psychiatric hospitalization, and at plenty of other times as well. She and I maintained a strong and trusting relationship over the years. I believe it was a comfort to both of us that I remained available to her, even if we only met intermittently.

I described this scenario to Barbara because, after a period of over a year of relative stability with respect to her mental health, the young woman was slated to graduate from high school. This was an extraordinarily meaningful goal for her to achieve given the ways in which her academic aims had been derailed in the years prior. She had invited me to her graduation ceremony, and although in previous professional positions it had been expected that I would not socialize with clients outside of the specific context of the work, I was interested in making a decision informed by best practice and not simply as a parroting of prior, and substantively quite different, work environments. Barbara asked me intuitive and helpful questions, and ultimately supported my arrival at the decision to attend the graduation of this young woman. I was grateful to Barbara both because of her assistance in this matter and her willingness to recognize that while in her psychoanalytic therapy practice attendance at a graduation would be an inappropriate and dangerous crossing of necessary therapeutic boundaries, in this case it was very different because it required paying attention to different types of boundaries in order to assess the options and understand their meaning for my client. Barbara seems to possess an innate ability to step outside of the existing framework of her own specific professional mandates in order to most successfully, holistically, and efficaciously supervise a clinician.

Integration of clinical wisdom into supervision

Barbara introduced role play into her work with my team, encouraging the case managers to interact with her and enact scenarios that involved clients in order to gain insight using techniques beyond simply conversing with a supervisor about a dynamic or situation. Having the opportunity to observe Barbara's instruction with my team has been invaluable to me, and I have often been able to integrate new techniques into my own supervision of staff. One role play that I observed and particularly appreciated involved a case manager whom I supervise describing to Barbara a scenario in which one of her clients, a woman nearly 80 years of age, was struggling. Her great-grandson's girlfriend had "taken over" the home by moving in with her four children and was not responsive to the established rules and culture of the home that the client had previously maintained for decades.

After the case manager had described the familial interrelationships and dynamics, Barbara suggested a role play in which the case manager played the client and Barbara played the case manager. Barbara proceeded to utilize psychodynamic techniques and practices within the case management relationship in order to facilitate problem-solving with respect to the home and family dynamics. Barbara's expert ability to weave clinical wisdom into any interaction—including those outside of the classical and boundaried therapeutic relationship, and even for direct staff who do not have a specific clinical educational background—is remarkable and shone through much of the work we did together. Ultimately, this modeled for me the ways in which I could do the same for my own team in our one-on-one supervision sessions.

Conclusion

My work with Barbara has had a monumental impact on my work as a therapist and supervisor. Not only have I been able to watch her strategically supervise my own team, which has strengthened my work as a supervisor, but her offering of support and space to me for the express purpose of exploring appropriate boundaries (given the community-embedded quality of my work) has forever shifted my own practice as well as the very landscape of the community-driven work within the organization.

Barbara's support and supervision has such importance, not only because of the specific content she has incorporated and as a supervisor of others but also because of her drawing upon her expertise outside of the scheduled monthly sessions. I have always been deeply struck by Barbara's willingness to speak with me and offer concrete input at a moment's notice—from early on in our relationship, she advised me to call her whenever needed. Barbara's incredible modeling of supervisory care and attention has improved my skills in this area considerably. Since it is not a formal board requirement, few organizations are hiring clinical supervisors for their senior clinicians (LCSWs) once they obtain their clinical license. However, supervisory support imbues the work with care, depth, resources, a sounding board for ethical practice, and someone with one degree of separation from the content who can really guide a clinician to an understanding that would be difficult to arrive at independently given the proximity to the situation. I feel lucky to work within a profession that values and recognizes the importance of supervision, albeit somewhat disproportionately for those without clinical licensures. It is a commodity that I believe is worth fighting for within the field and ought to be normalized and invested in. I am grateful to Barbara for revealing so much of this to me in our work together, and I dream of a social work profession in which all clinicians have access to a similar source of clinical support.

Note

1 All identifying information has been disguised to protect the privacy of the client/patient. Any resemblance to actual persons, living or dead, is purely coincidental.

Chapter 8

Supervision across disciplines and theoretical orientations

Allison Abrams

Introduction

My initial encounter with supervision took place during my first-year field placement within a transitional residential facility for formerly homeless, substance-abusing men. As a social work intern, a large part of my job was to help clients secure adequate housing, employment, and other basic needs. My supervisor was the director of the residential facility. Her education and expertise lay in the administrative rather than the clinical sphere of social work. Much of our supervision time—when we actually did get to meet, barring any crises or administrative priorities—was focused on the more immediate and practical issues that arose in the sessions and less on psychoanalytic exploration.

My first "real" psychoanalytic supervision experience would not occur until years later. After graduating with a Master of Social Work (MSW) degree and completing multiple fellowships, I decided to enroll in the Contemporary Freudian Society's (CFS) Psychodynamic Psychotherapy Program, with the ultimate goal of moving into private practice. Given the limited focus on psychoanalytic therapy in graduate school, I was aware that I would need more in-depth training in order to be an effective clinician.

As first-year students at the CFS, our supervisors were assigned to us. I learned that my supervisor would be Dr. Barbara Stimmel, a senior training analyst and former president of the Freudian Society. As a relatively new clinician, the idea of working with someone like Barbara was intimidating. Would she think I was a good clinician, or that I was even ready to start a private practice? Those were some of the insecurities that I would carry with me into our first supervision session.

First impression

My immediate impression upon meeting Barbara confirmed my feelings of trepidation, and a slight case of "imposter syndrome" swiftly kicked into gear. An intimidating presence at first glance, Barbara did not appear to be like the touchy-feely, motherly supervisory figures I had encountered earlier in my social work career, those with whom I had enjoyed many lunches and coffee breaks, sharing stories and eventually forming friendships. Instead, she was a no-nonsense, get down to business, consummate professional. Her office was nondescript, with low lighting, blank walls devoid of diplomas or other identifying information, the standard therapist's armchair, a bookcase overflowing with psychoanalytic literature, and one classical psychoanalytic couch. Did anyone even use those anymore, I wondered? And finally, just above her chair, hung a large photo of Sigmund Freud.

A lesson in transference

When I was growing up, I had a teacher who was notorious for her stern demeanor and penchant for yelling at children. As a shy and quiet kid, I was naturally intimidated and made sure not to do anything to upset her, lest she yell and embarrass me in front of my classmates. When I first met Barbara, there was something in her manner that triggered that familiar feeling from way back in my elementary school days. On some unconscious level, and in the most subtle way, she reminded me of that teacher. My unconscious self had mistaken Barbara's seriousness for something other than what it was. As I got to know her, however, I was quickly reminded of the faultiness of first impressions, that things—just like people—are not always as they first appear. To be able to differentiate between biased and sometimes distorted perceptions and objective truths is exactly what we want to teach our patients. We each bring our own life histories, and thus perspectives, into our interactions. Many times, these perceptions are inaccurate and, as such, the source of much interpersonal conflict. By making the unconscious conscious, we build ego strength and thus our ability to reality test. In other words, when we become sufficiently psychologically mature, we are able to build healthier relationships with others as well as with ourselves. As I got to know Barbara, it became clear that my immediate impression of her was primarily a transferential reaction and certainly a distorted one.

"First and foremost, the therapeutic relationship is unlike any other relationship."

Despite years spent in my own therapy and the therapeutic work that I had done thus far in my career as a social worker, as I embarked on the journey of psychoanalytic training, I wanted to go back to the drawing board and gain a more concrete understanding of this seemingly mystical process we call "psychotherapy." So, my first question to Barbara was: "What, really, is the aim of our work?" She broke it down for me in simple layman's terms, free of psychoanalytic jargon, which is the way she would teach me to speak to my patients: "We want to take the past out of the present." She explained that as we help our patients better understand the past, the less control it will have over their present. "You want to find out their world; their idiosyncrasies. Listen, follow, stay with them, and while doing so, you will begin to understand what is connected to what. How the past is connected to the present."

Whenever I approached Barbara with a general question about the work, she rarely answered without first asking about the particular patient to whom I was referring, thus reminding me that when it comes to the human condition, there is no one-size-fits-all formula. Each patient has their own unique history, story, and way of seeing the world. To quote Anaïs Nin: "We don't see things as they are, we see them as we are."

"We have to teach our patients how to be patients."

Barbara explained to me that we are essentially teaching our patients how to be patients—not in a didactic way, but rather by showing them how our minds, as therapists, work. She explained:

> The goal is to get them to start thinking about things the way that you do. You are inviting the patient to sit in your [the therapist's] chair, figuratively speaking, and to look at themselves with a critical eye and with curiosity, not judgment. You are helping them develop an observing ego.

She then gave the following example to illustrate her point:

> Imagine you take your child to see a movie, and there are some parts that the child finds scary. Maybe you have your arms around them, or they sit in your lap, and you watch together. Because you are not afraid, you are letting them know they do not have to be afraid. Slowly they may begin to uncover their eyes, finger by finger, to take a peek here and there, until they feel safe enough to uncover their eyes entirely.

For me, this description encapsulates the entire essence of the work. By helping our patients develop an observing ego, we are helping them increase their capacity for self-awareness, and thus the ability to have more control over both their internal and external worlds.

Self-disclosure

"A therapy session is not a conversation. It is work."

When a patient asks the therapist a personal question, Barbara explained, it is important to keep in mind that it is not the answer to the question that matters; it is the patient's motivation for asking it. It is the fantasies around what that answer may be. By answering right away, Barbara explained, we are cutting short the process of further exploration:

> Learn to listen more. Bring it back to the patient. The questions that they pose help us understand. Ask them what it feels like to not know

> anything about you. Get them to associate. Say, "Let's look at the central question. Rather than answer it, I can help *you* answer it." Focus on the question itself, not the answer. It is often too easy for therapy to become a casual exchange. You do not have to chitchat.

Developing confidence as a therapist

It was shortly after I began my work with Barbara that I opened my private practice. Having previously worked primarily in mental health clinics and social service agencies, the prospect of venturing out on my own was daunting. I would be leaving behind the safety of community mental health, where supports were readily available in the immediate vicinity from direct supervisors, program directors, and peers. In private practice, however, I would essentially be on my own. Admittedly, I had some doubts about my readiness to take this next step in my professional career. Ultimately, Barbara's support and encouragement played a large part in my decision to begin the practice when I did. She believed that I could do it, that I was a "good-enough therapist"—and if Barbara believed it, then perhaps it was true.

Barbara was there to guide me as I set up the logistics of my practice. "You must become firm in how you structure your practice," she informed me. She said:

> Once you know, "This is how I work, this is not how I work," or "This is how I conduct my practice," you can feel freer to stay firm. Do not have a rule per patient; rather, have a general clinical rule. Be confident in saying, "This is what I can offer." You don't have to accept every referral sent your way.

Hearing this from Barbara was a source of relief. As an experienced and competent clinician, I had earned the right to take charge of my practice, which made the work more satisfying and certainly more rewarding. Barbara validated this for me.

"You are the expert."

At times, when I expressed feelings of insecurity around my competence as a therapist, Barbara was quick to reassure me and remind me why our patients come to us. "You are the authority—not with a capital 'A.' Not in an *authoritarian* way. Rather, in a more benevolent way. More Nancy Pelosi." This made me laugh, and it also hit home. Moreover, she said:

> We are the experts. I am using this tone, not to be obnoxious or sound like I'm so smart. But to remind you that they have come to you for your expertise. Both the therapist and the patient are each supplying a different piece of the work. Your role is as someone who can help them understand

themselves better. To offer your knowledge, your expertise. That is why they come to you.

"Some of the best therapists ..."

Barbara once told me, "What makes some of the best therapists really good is their comfort with the 'sadistic' part of therapy." A sadistic therapist? That sounded like an oxymoron to me, but Barbara explained:

> Sadistic in the sense that the patient may experience you as withholding at times. When someone is sitting across from you and they are in pain, our natural, human instinct would be to comfort them, perhaps go over and hug them, for example. Something in a more tangible way. We do not do that, and to a patient, and to you, that may feel like you are being withholding. What is important to remember is that simply being there with them, listening to them, [and] tolerating whatever is coming up for them is enormously helpful. You're not there to lull your patients, to soothe them. Yes, people come to us to feel better, but sometimes you have to feel worse before you can feel better.

When styles clash

Early in my work with Barbara, I was still forming my identity as a therapist and developing a working style that felt comfortable to me. I do not believe in a one-size-fits-all type of treatment. Rather, I see the value of learning and working with multiple modalities, from cognitive behavioral therapy to mindfulness-based therapy to psychoanalytic psychotherapy—all of which I incorporate into my work today. Barbara, on the other hand, is a staunch Freudian. So, how could we navigate this schism in our theoretical and clinical leanings and thus resolve the discrepancies in our working styles?

I had my questions about the reality of asking patients to participate in psychoanalysis four or five times per week in today's modern world. Given their constraints in terms of time, finances, and managed care, how realistic would it be to expect patients to come in multiple times per week? Barbara had her questions about my use of weekly psychotherapy (which on rare occasions was sometimes less than weekly). This would become a topic of discussion during many supervision sessions. "Don't worry if you are not doing 'psychoanalysis,'" Barbara assured me. Rather,

> It is the way that you are thinking that is important and is what you will apply to the work. Yes, you have less time together, so there will be less free association; however, you will still follow their train of thought and judiciously make interpretations. No matter what form the therapy takes, in a successful treatment, the patient will come to identify with your way

> of thinking and be able to look at themselves and think about things the way that you do.

"Less than weekly therapy is not therapy."

This was Barbara's response when I described my flexibility with patients. I worked with people who traveled often and therefore were not able to attend therapy on a regular basis. Believing that it would be better for them to see me occasionally than not at all, I saw some of these patients on an as-needed basis. Sometimes they came in bi-monthly and sometimes even less often. When I heard Barbara say that this way of working was not "therapy," I became upset. Was she undermining the work that I had been doing with my patients—work that I believed was significant and impactful? She explained that this was not a judgment but rather a way of thinking about the frame. Eventually, I would come to understand and agree with her way of thinking, and I changed my practice accordingly. Intuitively, I knew that working with patients on an ad hoc or less than weekly basis was causing me frustration and making the work less satisfying. I now see patients at a minimum of once per week and sometimes, when possible, more than once per week. I have come to understand the significance of frequency as a catalyst for a deeper treatment and therapeutic relationship.

When I spoke with Barbara about my cases, it occurred to me that I often left out the cognitive and behavioral part of the work that I did with patients, such as helping them reframe their negative thought patterns in order to look at their core schemas and self-beliefs and ultimately change how they speak to themselves. Classical Freudians, on the other hand, tend to focus primarily on unconscious processes and childhood history. I understand the value of this and certainly incorporate it into my work; however, I also believe that modalities such as the ones described above can significantly further the treatment. Both are essential to healing. But how would I explain this to Barbara? Would she eschew my way of working or criticize the choices I made in my sessions? During one supervision session, I brought this up. Not surprisingly, she was receptive:

> Let's see if we can combine them. Let's see if we can extend the reframing to what you and the patient can do together. A cognitive therapeutic task always involves the therapist. Rather than assigning a task from the seat of the expert, even though you are the expert, suggest that you reframe [it] together. You could say, "If *we* could look at the behavior together, perhaps *we* can consider different ways of thinking about it." (Use we rather than you. You are doing this work together.) "I think we can look at those behaviors and see how they affect how you feel about yourself."

As I pondered this, it occurred to me once again that I did not have to follow the same exact formula as my supervisor, and that I could have my own way of working. Just as patients are individuals on their own personal journey toward growth, so too are therapists in finding and formulating our own professional identities. Ultimately, there is no right or wrong answer; nor is there one strict way of working. Every therapist, just like every supervisor, will come to develop their own working style.

Confrontation

One day, Barbara brought up my tendency to bend the structure at times, for example, changing my schedule to accommodate patients' schedules, even when it inconvenienced me. I thought that I was being compassionate, that I was facilitating the therapeutic process by being open and flexible with my rules. "Bullshit," Barbara said. Before I had a chance to respond, she followed this up with:

> I mean that in the best of ways. You may feel like you are helping by being so accommodating, but what you are really doing is enabling. By inconveniencing yourself, you are not doing anyone any favors. You are only risking resentment. Yes, you must think about their needs, but at the same time, you must consider your needs as well. When discussing [the] schedule, for example, it's not just about what will work for the patient, but what will work for the both of you. You are modeling healthy boundaries and self-care.

She pointed to the example of our own supervisor–supervisee interaction when we were negotiating our supervision schedule. When I specifically asked for a time later in the day, she was considerate of my needs and accommodated me when—and only when—it was feasible for her to do so, but without compromising her own needs, and thus preventing any resentment on either side. She helped me understand the difference between being a compassionate therapist and "deforming the frame." There is a delicate balance between being considerate and having boundaries (and therefore reliability). By participating with the patient in acting out (disregarding boundaries), I am actually robbing them of the opportunity to structure their life or to be reliable to themselves. Barbara said:

> Again, therapy is not like any other relationship. It is not helpful to keep meeting all of their needs all of the time. Keep myself in the mix of needs being met. It must work for me too. Be clear on what your "rules" are and confident on what your policy is. Let patients run around them. Let them "act out." We learn about them through their behaviors as much as through their verbal communication.

She explained that I am there to understand the actions of my patients, not to stop them. If I undo what is happening, then I am being "intrusive." I must let them play out what they need to play out. For example, if a patient forgets about a session, I should let them forget. Not coming in is something. It is their psychology. "Acting out" is not a negative, she explained. Instead of talking, it is another way of telling me something. It is just another source of information. My aim is not to change my patients; it is to help them become aware of their behaviors so they can choose their behaviors consciously. I do not necessarily want to stop the behavior; I want to analyze it and to use it as a cue.

The irony suddenly hit me. Many of the clients with whom I was working at the time were struggling with boundary setting. I was helping them understand their codependent behavior and patterns of placing others' needs before their own, which inevitably gave rise to resentment and ultimately burnout. Yet there I was, doing exactly the same, all the while believing that I was being helpful. Barbara said, "You are not a caretaker. It is their life and you are not there to 'fix it.' Let them play out what they need to play out, help them look at the consequences and discuss." This, of course, would not only positively affect the work, but it would also make a significant difference in how I felt while doing the work.

Building trust in the supervisory relationship

During one supervision session, I was describing a patient who had, according to Barbara, violated my physical space.[1] As the patient was describing an email he had received, he suddenly rose from the couch, walked around my chair, and stood over my shoulder as he showed me the email on his phone. It was a behavior not unlike others he had displayed in previous sessions. Barbara asked me if I read the email. Hesitantly, I told her that I had. This was a mistake, she informed me. But she quickly followed up by reassuring me that mistakes are not only OK, but also opportunities to learn. She explained that by reading the email as the patient had asked, I was participating in the boundary violation that was taking place:

> You are caught up in an enactment which must be addressed. Don't read the email. Instead, offer that he read it to you. But also explore his desire for you to read it. He crossed a boundary. He did not respect your personal space. This is a behavior he displays in his other relationships, which causes him difficulties. Therefore, it must be addressed in the room.

In that moment, was Barbara confronting *me* indirectly? Was she telling *me* that I had just crossed a physical boundary by enacting the interaction with my patient? Perhaps my anxiety about the patient feeling criticized was a projection of my own sensitivity to Barbara's feedback as a form of criticism. It would be wise to "confront" Barbara with this. In the spirit of becoming more comfortable with confrontation, I decided to ask her. If I could not be honest with my supervisor, could I ask in good faith that my patients be honest with me? If I am not comfortable with conflict, how will I be able to effectively manage the conflict that will inevitably arise in therapy?

"Barbara, did you feel that I violated your boundaries when I just got out of my seat and stood beside you?" With genuine compassion, she replied, "No, that was very different. I knew what you were doing. You asked me if you could show me how the patient acted." Hearing this, I was relieved. Having confronted her, and her receiving it, we were able to move forward. Then I knew that I could confront my supervisor without fear of her retaliating or thinking of me as a less than competent therapist. I knew that I could trust her.

Trust is an essential ingredient in the supervisor–supervisee relationship, just as it is in the therapist–patient relationship and ultimately in all of our relationships. Here in supervision, I had a safe space where I could practice open communication and healthy confrontation without the fear of irreparably rupturing the relationship. This is exactly what we want for all of our patients.

As difficult as it may have been at first, I realized that if I am to ask my patients to leave their comfort zones, then I must be able to step out of my own and be comfortable with the uncomfortable. Intimate relationships are not devoid of occasional conflict. Confronting these conflicts or ruptures is at the core of this work, after all. There will inevitably be bumps in the road as there are in all relationships—even in the supervisory relationship. Psychological growth involves addressing these bumps. If we can teach our patients to do this in the treatment room, then hopefully they will be able to do the same in their other relationships. Similarly, if we as therapists want to help our patients resolve conflict, then we must be able to do the same, especially with our supervisors. In fact, after our own therapy, supervision is one of the best places to practice.

The chaotic patient

One session, I began by asking Barbara to read an email that I had received from a patient whom I had been seeing since he was an adolescent. The first thing Barbara asked was why did I want her to read it? Her follow-up question was why did the patient want me to read it? I had not thought about this. What is the patient inducing in me that I am now enacting with my supervisor? The patient wants me to understand him better. Similarly, I want to be able to explain the patient better to Barbara, which I was having a hard time doing. I had always found both the case and the patient to be too complicated to articulate or present in a cohesive manner, which is why I had avoided bringing it up until that moment. As I had anticipated, I found myself stumbling as I presented the case and was unable to answer Barbara's continual line of questioning. Barbara said,

> I have 20 questions for you about this patient, most of which you are unable to answer. You are showing me, in here, what it is like for you in the room with the patient. You are lost at sea.

She continued, "There is a parallel process happening. He is showing you what it was like for him growing up." Barbara advised me to get a better history, even though I had been working with the patient for several years. She said that it is always OK to go back.

> Take a pause. Take him by the shoulders, metaphorically speaking, and say "Let's stop and try to get a better picture so that I can figure out how to help you." So that you could get a hold of the steering wheel. That is why they are coming to us. We are the ones who know how to steer the boat. Otherwise they would stay on their own boats! You need to contain him. Let him know that over the next few sessions, you will be asking a lot of questions in order to better understand his "story." Do not use the term "history." That is too clinical. Explore with him his tendency to be disorganized at times in his presentation. Perhaps it is a way to keep people at a distance. Get a more cohesive, structured story so that you can bring in and present a more cohesive case to me.

That is exactly what I would go on to do. And once I was better able to understand and present a cohesive case, as she had done so many times previously, Barbara effectively helped me to navigate yet another bumpy journey on the path to exploring human complexities.

When the supervisor makes a mistake

One day, I sat patiently in the waiting room, waiting for Barbara to emerge so we could start our supervision session. Fifteen minutes had passed since the scheduled start time, and she still had not arrived. That was when my anxiety began to kick in. This was not like Barbara. If she was ever late, it was rarely more than a couple of minutes. One of my first thoughts was that she might have forgotten about our appointment. I wondered if I should knock on her door. What if she was in a session or on an important phone call and I interrupted with my impatient knocking? But if I did not knock on her door, how long would I have to sit and wait? Eventually, Barbara emerged and apologized. She had the wrong time written down and thought that we were meeting 30 minutes later than we were scheduled. She expressed her embarrassment. She even used the "enactment" as an example in the supervision that day. She used the example of her own embarrassment about being late to describe the embarrassment that a patient may feel when making a mistake. She brought the elephant into the room and not only talked about it, but also used it as part of the work to serve as a wonderful example of how we as therapists should handle our own mishaps with patients. What I learned was that I should own it when I do something clumsy, to say, "I'm sorry, yes, I could have handled that better," and invite the patient to look at it with me rather than ignore it.

Coincidentally, or perhaps fortuitously, a few weeks after this supervision session, I ended up double-booking two patients in my practice. When both patients showed up at the same time, I was at first confused and then embarrassed. "How could I have made such a careless mistake?" I asked myself. But then I remembered what had occurred in that session with Barbara. She owned her mistake. She admitted that she was human, as we all are, and she took accountability for her actions. If it had not been supervision but rather a therapy session, we would have processed what had taken place and explored my feelings around it (e.g., my anxiety while waiting for her and my thoughts of being forgotten), which is just what I did eventually with both of those patients. It turned out that this "rupture" actually ended up deepening the work with both patients, as ruptures often do, and brought further trust into the therapeutic relationship. I believe the same occurred in my relationship with Barbara.

The suicidal patient

"Your role as a therapist is profound, but it is limited."

In one supervision session, I was discussing a patient who had a history of suicidal ideation and one suicide attempt when he was younger. Discussing a recent session in which he had expressed suicidal ideation, I asked Barbara, "When a patient presents with suicidal ideation, how much of the session do you devote to the issue of basic safety (as opposed to psychoanalyzing the cause)?" "Almost all of it!" she exclaimed, explaining:

> The first order of business is making sure he is connected to a psychiatrist. You have to know what your limits are as a therapist. If you were a cardiologist and your patient was diagnosed with cancer, you would send them to an oncologist, you would not treat them yourself. That is not your expertise. In addition to the patient's safety, you also have to be safe. If anything ever happened, you would never forgive yourself.

I asked if she had ever worked with a suicidal patient, and she replied:

> No, I don't work with suicidal patients, but I have had many colleagues who have had the unfortunate experience of losing a patient. It is devastating. Of course, you want to make sure that you have done everything that is in your power—within the limits of what you can do. Ask yourself, what are my limits? To what extent can I help? What is my skill set? Where do my skills begin and end? You are assessing the distress that the patient is in emotionally. But you are not assessing medication.

A strong proponent of self-determination, I believe that when it comes to medication and other such decisions, it is ultimately the patient's choice. However, as Barbara explained, if a patient is describing suicidal thoughts, especially with a detailed plan, it should be made a requirement that in order to work together, they must also be in the care of a psychiatrist, or, at the very least, have a psychiatric evaluation, allowing another expert to provide an opinion. Then I would know that I was not alone. Barbara insisted that I should not be sitting alone with this. She said, "It is not fair to you. The fact that you had the impulse to call me after the session is a clear marker that you needed someone else to get involved. He needs an evaluation!"

I was aware that my own hesitancy mirrored that of the patient's. By explaining it to me in this way, Barbara helped me gain confidence in making a clinical decision.

> You can say, "It is not a command. It is an expectation. In order for us to continue working together. To help you in ways that I cannot. These thoughts have come up in the past and I can see how distressing it must be. Medication can take the edge off, thus making our work together easier and provide you some relief so that we can work on the underlying issues." We want to help the patient cope. After all, if a patient is unable to function, the psychotherapeutic work will not be as productive. Some things that you can do to help are increasing the frequency of sessions, come up with a safety plan, and be available for emergencies. But that is about all.

This all made sense and was what I knew intuitively, but having Barbara confirm my intuition bolstered my confidence in managing a difficult situation. The patient ended up being seen by a psychiatrist and was started on medication.

On termination: endings and losses

"The loss of a love object is a major source of anxiety for human beings."

Unfortunately, most therapists do not terminate "properly." No one likes talking about endings or separations. It is easy to talk about the beginning and middle phases of therapy, but the ending should be treated as just as significant as the beginning—perhaps even more so. After all, you and the patient have been through so much together. Ultimately, we want our patients to be able to leave us. We want them to depend on us—in a healthy way—so that they can eventually leave us. It is oxymoronic, but that is what therapy is about—bringing them closer so that they can leave us. But how do we know if a patient is ready for termination? I wanted to know, so I asked Barbara.

> When deciding whether to terminate or not, you must look at the *character* of the patient. Has the character changed? Is the behavior different? For example, have they stopped fighting with people, have their relationships improved? Has the patient "worked through?" Working through is the giving up of the unconscious fantasy. Have they accessed the forbidden wish so that it no longer has the same motivational power? We are neurotic because of how much we try to suppress the unacceptable feelings. Ego-mastering is learning to tolerate this. To accept the heartache of the unfulfilled wish. Our goal is to strengthen the ego to become the agent of our own

life, to become less impulse-ridden. Analysis is about strengthening the ego to quell the power of the impulses and mediate between the superego and the id. We help the ego flourish to be the stronger structure.

Concluding thoughts

Despite our differing clinical styles and, to some extent, clinical beliefs, Barbara and I were able to make the supervisory relationship work. Somehow, we would adapt Barbara's way of working as a classical Freudian psychoanalyst to my more contemporary once-weekly psychotherapy. I learned from her, and I would like to believe that she also learned from me in the same way that we learn from our patients.

Our patients come to us from various cultural backgrounds, each seeing the world through a different lens. Ultimately, we all come from the same human family. Supervisors and supervisees do not necessarily have to come from the same school of thought or cultural background to learn from one another. Communication, mutual trust, and respect are the key ingredients of an effective supervisory relationship regardless of discipline, style, or cultural background. When we work together to understand one another and remain open to learning, we are likely to have a successful and rewarding supervision experience.

What I have shared in this chapter is but a fraction of what I have learned throughout my work with Barbara. Just as important as the wisdom that Barbara has imparted to me is what I have learned through the relationship with Barbara itself. For example, I have learned not always to trust first impressions, and that there are many different ways that one can be supportive and helpful. And, just as it is with therapy, I learned that the most important factor in supervision is the relationship between the supervisor and supervisee rather than the technique itself. We must ask ourselves, "Does the patient feel safe, heard, and seen?" And we must do the same with supervision.

I am confident that my work with Barbara has played a significant role in my growth as a clinician. It has helped shape my professional identity, informed my work with patients, and influenced the way that I run my practice today. It is my hope that all therapists and mental health professionals might be so lucky as to find a supervisor whom they trust and with whom they can embark on this rewarding journey of psychotherapy.

Note

1 All identifying information has been disguised to protect the privacy of the client/patient. Any resemblance to actual persons, living or dead, is purely coincidental.

Chapter 9

Two detectives working on a case

Liat Shklarski

Introduction

I started working with Barbara six years ago as part of a mandatory supervision requirement for a postgraduate psychoanalytic psychotherapy program I attended. My colleague, Allison Abrams, who was my classmate and had been in supervision with Barbara in her first year of the program, recommended that I contact her. She conveyed to me that Barbara was a very smart clinician and had a strong "analytic" orientation. I was told that Barbara was a "mini Freud" and that I would like her very direct style. This captured my interest because I appreciate straightforward, open conversation and receiving feedback.

At that time, I was in my early clinical career. I had graduated with a master's in social work four years earlier and was a newly licensed clinical social worker (LCSW). I was working in community mental health, providing one-on-one psychotherapy counseling, and I was in the very early stages of pursuing my PhD. I remember being very passionate about developing my clinical skills and understanding the theory that I was trying to apply in practice. Most importantly, I remember how insecure I was about my clinical work, my identity as a clinician, and the fact that English was my second language. I felt that I did not always understand everything, and definitely was not yet accustomed to American culture.

My first few sessions in supervision with Barbara: do I like her style?

My insecurities followed me to my first meeting with Barbara. Meeting a senior analyst—a psychologist—was intimidating for me; I was afraid to be judged. I remember the moment that we met. I was wearing jeans and a blouse. Barbara escorted me into her office, which was relatively dark. In the room, there was a very noticeable analytic couch, a signed photo of Sigmund Freud, plenty of books, and two armchairs. To add to that, there was construction going on outside the office, and the noise was incredibly distracting. My insecurities were growing, and I was certain that Barbara would not be able to understand anything I said in my broken English.

Barbara was quick to apologize for the noise, and dove right into the supervision hour by asking: "What kind of work do you do?" I was very proud of my work in community mental health, and I was ready to talk about it. But then came a very uncomfortable (for me) question about my clothing. "This is what you wear to work?" she asked. I could not see the connection between the two, and I became very defensive. Internally, I was ready to leave and never come back. I felt hurt and judged. What could my clothing possibly have to do with my clinical work with patients?

Reflecting back on that moment, I realize that I may have interpreted her comment through a lens of professional insecurity relating to my strong need to defend my professional identity as a social worker. Barbara was a practicing psychologist, and I was worried that she was looking down on me as a social worker.

So why did I end up going back to meet with her again? I definitely returned with the mission of protecting and advocating for my profession. But I also did so because that first conversation I had with Barbara was very different from any other conversation I had had with supervisors in the past; she was very direct and very motivated to help me. I could see that she was genuinely interested in what I had to say.

In previous chapters, we addressed the power dynamic that exists in the supervisory relationship. Hierarchy is part of the student–teacher supervisory relationship; but I want to highlight that, as supervisees, we also have a degree of power. We should dare to broach conversations with our supervisors when we feel uncomfortable, which brings me back to my second session with Barbara. Looking back, I am happy that I decided to discuss my feelings with her and continue the supervisory relationship instead of quitting.

In our second meeting, I started by sharing with her how I felt about the questions she had asked the last time. Barbara did not blink, and quickly explained that by understanding what I wear to work, she can get an idea of the setting of my clinical practice. She provided me with a thorough explanation of why she needed to learn about the nature of my work, my clinical style, and the setting in order to effectively supervise me. She did not get caught up in my professional insecurities, and instead jumped right into creating a "working space" for us.

Her explanation made sense; she had to understand my professional identity as a clinician in order to best serve me as my supervisor. More importantly, her explanation made me feel safer; she was confident and provided a very professional explanation that made me sit back and begin to let go of my insecurities. I felt as if I were in good hands and that she (as my potential supervisor) was genuinely trying to help me advance my clinical work by prioritizing my agenda and adapting her supervision to suit my professional needs. To this day, I still do not know if she is even aware that her initial line of questioning about my clothing and my work in community mental health inspired my internal exploration and reflection on my work and professional development.

In fact, supervision was the catalyst for my departure from the community mental health clinic. When I met with Barbara, I would share my frustration with the rules and restrictions of community mental health that prevented me from doing the clinical work I was eager to do. A mere two months after I started my supervisory relationship with Barbara, I decided to enter private practice. In this short time, Barbara had already instilled in me a sense of having the power to effect change, saying, "When you are not content, you need to make changes; the agency is not going to change." Since then, I have carried this idea with me in both my professional and personal life.

The supervisory relationship is not just about clinical development; I perceive it as a working relationship. At times, the supervisor takes on other professional roles such as those of mentor, coach, and teacher. Barbara had never told me that I should leave the clinic, but she invited me to think about it from a different perspective and gave me the confidence to act on it.

Throughout my career, I have valued the supervisory relationship and have always been in clinical supervision outside of the agency I have worked for. I appreciate alternative viewpoints and the opportunity to learn how to navigate sessions in different ways. Supervision has always been a remarkable learning opportunity for me—almost like uncovering new clues when solving a mystery. It is an ongoing feeling that something that I was previously unaware of is being brought to the surface by the supervisor, which means that I can then move forward with my patient's treatment.

I often ask myself why I keep returning to supervision and why in particular I keep coming back to Barbara. When looking for a supervisor, one should see the supervisor–supervisee interaction as a relationship. My experience of the supervisory relationship has helped shape the way I understand my patients and think about their problems. It may have started as a consultation about one particular patient, but it has reformed how I think clinically. Barbara's ideas, questions, and way of thinking about my patients' problems have stayed with me when I am in the room with them and when I am supervising and teaching my colleagues.

About this chapter

Over the next few pages, I am going to present an overview of more than a year of supervision sessions with Barbara in which we discussed a single case that was challenging for me. Throughout the chapter, I will almost equate the supervisory experience to that of two detectives working a case together and trying to solve it. In this particular case, supervision helped me navigate difficult moments in the therapeutic process, helped me understand why the patient acted in certain ways, and gave me guidance on how to terminate the therapeutic relationship.[1] I have chosen to subdivide the material into a series of questions and answers, mainly because these are the questions that Barbara would often ask me or questions that I would ask her. I will conclude with some important elements that shaped my supervisory relationship with Barbara in the hopes of giving the readers insight into what their effective supervisory relationships might look like.

The therapeutic work in conjunction with supervision

A few years ago, I was working with a woman in her mid-twenties. She had decided to pursue therapy because she was dissatisfied with her current life. In the beginning stages of my work with the patient, I did not think that I would need to consult with Barbara about this case. However, it became evident that I would need to when I found myself feeling stuck, bored, and frustrated both before and during sessions with the patient. Yet, I also had a lot of compassion for the patient; it almost felt like she was a child who was lost in the world and needed guidance. From time to time, I became curious about her and resisted the urge to Google her name to find out more information about her, her family, and who she was.

"Who is the patient in the world outside of the therapeutic relationship?"

I began to discuss the case in supervision mainly because I felt like no matter how I directed our sessions, the patient found ways to return to the fact that she needed to change her life but did not know how. Barbara's first question to me was one that I have always kept in mind since then. She asked,

> What is her history? Who is this person in the world? Do not just tell me demographics. Liat, you want to know about her parents, does she have siblings, relationships, where she went to school, her appearance, and her living situation.

She added, "How did she find you? Who referred her to you? Was it her idea to go to therapy?"

In hindsight, it was obvious. Of course, we have to know these things when we interact with our patients; but I was also skeptical about asking these questions because I knew that the patient was not going to give me the details. I shared my thoughts with Barbara and she reframed the question: "Why do you not know some of these things; or, why has the patient not shared those details?" Her new way of asking the question invited me to think differently about the patient and the relationship, which also assisted me in the conversation with the patient.

"What do we do when we find ourselves, as therapists, sometimes sitting in front of patients feeling that we cannot make meaning of their narratives?"

During my interactions with the patient, I often felt unsure about how to engage her, and I often wondered how she engaged me. It seemed that the conversation would not go deeper or further. The patient kept the conversation very superficial and left me wondering about her, her problems, and the solutions to her problems. It felt as if she was hoping that I would tell her what her problems were (as opposed to helping her work through the problems that she had identified) or tell her what to do in order to solve them.

I tried to ask fewer questions and to speak only when it was critical. As much as I tried, it did not work. I would remain silent and ask her to tell me more, to elaborate on her stories; and I would even reflect back and comment that her stories were vague and that I needed more information in order to help her figure out the root of her presented problem. But the answers I was given remained the same—they were still very vague and offered no new information.

Every week, I shared my frustrations with Barbara. In return, she would listen carefully and role play with me. She got stuck and was sometimes frustrated, and she used theory to describe and understand the character of the patient. I felt comfortable with Barbara, who had never made me feel that I was not doing a good job, and instead validated that the work was challenging. I appreciated that she had never let me feel as if I were doing something wrong, but explored the therapeutic relationship with me instead. She explained that we could understand the patient's interactions with me as resistance,[2] meaning that she had erected an unconscious barrier to learning more about herself, to letting me know more about her, and to actually finding a solution to her problem(s). At that point, I did not know enough about her resistance and why she was resisting; was she afraid to reveal some new information that would lead to change? If she effected change, what would happen? I reflect back on this time now and remember how hard it was to pick up on the resistance right away: on the one hand, she was attending therapy regularly and showing interest; but on the other hand, the treatment did not progress, no developments were made, and no future change was to be seen.

"How do we engage with vague stories therapeutically?"

The patient was engaging with me by either not providing information about her past or by providing vague descriptions of her life that made me both very curious and at times very frustrated. I went to Barbara feeling very perplexed. Yet again, I felt stuck, inadequate, and lacking in the skills required to help the patient. But I also felt empathy for the patient; I liked her, and I looked forward to seeing her. Barbara was always there to reassure me that I should be aware of my feelings toward my patients. When I felt stuck, Barbara became more active, and I never left a supervisory meeting with her feeling stuck, only more motivated to meet with the patient and explore new avenues.

In one of our sessions, Barbara made an important comment, which was that the client must have been acting with me the same way that she acted with her parents, siblings, and other important people in her life. Barbara made me think outside of the box, and I realized that I was just like them.

The patient had been in treatment for almost a year already, and there had been no developments in either the therapeutic relationship or her life. "Liat, you need to insist on knowing more about who she is outside of the room," Barbara said. She explained that we always want to wonder whether the patient acts similarly in their other relationships. Does the patient repeat the same patterns in her relationship with me that she does in the relationships she has with the other significant people in her life? After all, if I am experiencing it, others must be experiencing it too.

What I appreciate the most about supervision is the ability to try out the suggestions in practice. In my sessions with the patient, I helped her wonder whether she replicates her relationship with her parents with me. I thought to myself that once we were both aware of that, we could look at it together and try to understand why she replicated those relationships in that way. Nevertheless, she kept minimizing any interpretation that I would make about the similarities between her relationships. I remember wondering if I had not explained myself well—was there a language barrier that prevented her from understanding me?

The detective work continued week after week; but Barbara did not give up, and was trying to understand the patient's emotional and physical presence when she was in the room with me. The patient usually appeared anxious, did not make eye contact, and often apologized. "Why is she anxious when she sits with you?" Barbara asked. "Who does she want you to be? (What relationship figure do you symbolize?)" Maybe she feared that I would lose interest, become impatient with her stagnation, and leave her. After all, from time to time, I did get impatient—or at least I felt like I wanted to yell at her. But Barbara had another thought. Maybe she was afraid that I would challenge her to the point that she would have to come to terms with the fact that she was *actively* behaving passively in her personal and professional life. Barbara suggested that I become more aware of my reactions, behaviors, and feelings toward the patient and eventually bring this up to the patient. It crossed my mind that I felt manipulated by the patient; but how was I going to tell her that she was not doing any work in therapy and that simply attending therapy was not enough?

At that point, I remembered a helpful tool that can be used in supervision—asking for guidance on how the supervisor would address such a problem with a patient. I simply asked, "If you were sitting in the room with the patient, what would you say?" Barbara was happy to answer while I took notes, but she also stressed, "Liat, find your own language, your way of saying it." I appreciated her ability to see me as a separate person in that instance.

I came to terms with the fact that I was caught in an enactment of my patient's relationships with others in her life.[3] The client wanted to let me know what it was like for her to be the daughter of her parents. I needed to stop and reflect. Did the patient act with resistance because she wanted to teach me about her feelings in her intimate relationships? Everyone told her what to do, second-guessed her, and controlled her; she felt that she had no choice, and, as a result, she stagnated. This dynamic was re-enacted with me.

My awareness of what seemed like projective identification was profound in my relationship with the patient.[4] Once I understood that, I could relate to her experiences and *hopefully* help her make changes.

Like many of my patients, the patient would often ask me for advice and want me to tell her what to do. From time to time, I would fall into the "trap" and express my opinion. While I was wrong to do so, I was also feeling like we had reached an impasse. I had to figure out how we could stop that habit and also figure out why the habit had formed. Barbara suggested that I ask the patient: "If I told you what to do, would you really do it?" It was a good question for me to remember and ask in practice—I needed to slow down and get the patient to think and act on her own.

"Why do we continue to do things that are unhealthy? (What's in it for you?)"

At times, Barbara invited me to flip the script or simply look at the problem from a different perspective. How does the patient benefit from the situation? If I helped the patient look at a situation, relationship, or problem from another perspective, maybe we could work through the resistance or at least become conscious of certain information. In other words, what did she gain from stagnating in life? When Barbara asked those questions, I tried to imagine what the patient would say, but I did not know how to answer that for her. This was a good sign that I was being helped by Barbara. Oftentimes, we role play (I play the role of the patient), and once I get stuck and can no longer think of what the patient might say, I know that I have found a new strategy to try.

This question of *What's in it for you?* is something that I bring into my interactions with patients. I always invite them to try to understand their reasons for acting in a certain way. Barbara has taught me to understand the fear of a life change as a conflict between a wish and a fear. On the one hand, there is the wish to develop and grow, and, on the other hand, there is a sense that it is impossible. The conflict between my patient's wish and her fear had shut her down to the point that her life had become stagnant.

Barbara always emphasized the importance of understanding the patient's conflicts and dilemmas. In this case, she invited me to think out loud with the patient about the possible options and outcomes: "What will happen if you do X as opposed to Y?" and "It occurs to me that you keep doing something that you do not like or that causes you a lot of stress. Let's try to think together about what is preventing you from changing (or keeping you stagnant)." I remember leaving that supervision with Barbara feeling like I had won the lottery—I had the tools I needed to help the patient explore her resistance and reflect on some of her fears of change. In my mind, once we could figure that part out, we could start making changes. Unfortunately, yet again, my efforts were unsuccessful, and the patient kept going back to a place where every attempt to explore a potential change or a different outlook was blocked.

Barbara is often able to give an outsider's point of view when I am caught up in an interaction with a patient. The patient described her situation as impossible to overcome, when in fact she was actually solving her conflict by doing nothing. On the one hand, she wanted to change. On the other, she was afraid of it, so she kept on being dependent—that was her solution to the conflict of separation. I needed to be confident in my skills to help her see that she was actively making decisions to remain stagnant (after all, it is a decision) because either she did not want to change or she was not ready to change.

"What do we do when we feel ill-equipped to help our patients or we have exhausted all of our options?"

After many hours of supervision, I came to terms with the fact that the patient was not going to make the changes that she wished for. I felt defeated; I had exhausted all of the tools in my toolkit without seeing a change. With Barbara's help, I realized that the change would not come from the patient—it was up to me to make the changes in our relationship. It seemed as though the best solution would be for me to take action and change the framework of the treatment by initiating the termination process. Barbara was very supportive and seemed to agree with me. I believe that Barbara knew this was the only way to make a change, but I am glad that she did not push me or tell me what to do. Instead, she provided me with the time I needed to grow as a clinician and come to this conclusion on my own.

The rationale for the termination emphasized the fact that we were not really working therapeutically. The treatment is a mirror of the patient's life; she was stuck in her personal and professional life and we were stuck in the therapeutic relationship. Working through the termination for over two months was very painful. I was very much committed to working with the patient, but I also understood how important it was for us to make a change. We agreed on the date of our last appointment. Two weeks prior, the patient left a voicemail before our penultimate session and said that she would rather it be the final one instead. I was surprised, conflicted, and happy. I did not want to let her go, but knew I had to. I was glad that she prepared me for that so I could actually ask her more about the decision and comment on the fact that she was changing—for once, she had actively made a decision.

It is never too late to go back

As therapists, we usually attend supervision in between sessions with our patients. During the supervision hour, while processing earlier sessions that I have had with patients, I often feel as if I have missed opportunities in those sessions to make "profound" statements. Barbara has always reassured me that it is never too late to return to materials and make connections. She has helped build my self-esteem, and certainly reduced my anxiety about doing things correctly. I do not always need to say the right thing in the session; I can process it in supervision, understand the concept, and get back to the patient to make new connections later.

Using my personal experiences as a mother to think about my patients' internal lives

In the supervisory relationship, the sharing of personal experiences is inevitable. Barbara knows about my personal life—specifically, she knows about my multiple roles as a clinician, educator, scholar, mother, and partner. I will always appreciate and use her unique way of helping me understand my patients by relating to my experiences as a mother. Oftentimes, Barbara invites me to think about my role as a mother and my interactions with my own children in order to conceptualize how I should understand the unconscious parts of my patients and my own behaviors with them. Since it was very hard for me to terminate with the patient that I described in this chapter, an important moment in the supervisory relationship occurred when Barbara invited me to think of the ways I help my children develop a sense of independence. Suddenly, I realized that being conflicted about stopping the therapeutic work was similar to my role as a mother. On the one hand, I want my children to be dependent on me; but, on the other hand, it is my job to teach them to be self-sufficient, independent people. I had to remember that I needed to be the mother that I was to my children in my relationship with the patient as well—one who trusts herself as a parent and trusts her children as a result of that parenting.

Drawing on my personal life in supervision has helped me set clearer boundaries with patients who are intrusive or have borderline personality traits. I have to keep reminding myself that in their transference is the desire that I will be their caretaker or "take them home with me." However, in the work I have done with Barbara, there has been a great emphasis on learning how to protect myself and my special role as a mother to my own children, as well as how to protect the patient by reminding them that my power is limited and boundaries are necessary. Regardless of whether a patient might fantasize that I will do everything for them, like a "good" mother might do for her child, I can convey to them that while I am there for them, it is in a way that is different from how I am there for my own children.

Learn to live in peace with your supervisor: it is OK to have different approaches

So far, I have described a very peaceful supervisory relationship. However, many times our views have conflicted; I cannot always relate to or agree with what Barbara says. At first, I thought that since a senior and very gifted psychoanalyst was sitting in front of me, she must always be right. But my relationship with Barbara has taught me that we are very different. The differences in our characters, our clinical approaches, and our work with patients are things that we both need to accept. Barbara almost seems to enjoy the moments when I disagree with her. Her eyes light up and she becomes more curious. I find the back and forth to be stimulating, and it allows me to think differently about the clinical materials.

I encourage supervisees to explore their disagreements with their supervisors, confident in the knowledge that disagreement in a healthy supervisory relationship will always lead to a positive outcome. There were times that I did not agree with Barbara; sometimes it was my resistance to approach a problem with the patient, and sometimes it was because of our different styles and approaches. I have learned to be more open with Barbara about our different approaches. One example that comes to mind is in our communication with patients. While I allow for communication to take place over text, for Barbara, this is an unfamiliar concept. I used to hide it from Barbara, but the more confident I became, the more I was able to discuss our differences and not perceive them negatively. I recommend that supervisees share with their supervisors their clinical differences and definitely think that they should not be shy about it. This way, their exchanges with their supervisors become more authentic, and it allows the supervisee to experience significant growth.

Summary

I attribute a large part of my professional development to my supervision journey. Many times, I have met with Barbara unprepared, saying "I have nothing to talk about; nothing interesting is happening in the practice." Yet, she has always been able to make meaning of my reactions, stories, and interactions with patients. When I completed my PhD, I decided to "pay it forward" by supporting other clinicians' professional development, and I use many of Barbara's techniques and ideas—as well as her teaching/supervisory style—in my interactions with my own supervisees. It is gratifying for me to see their motivated faces when they leave the room feeling that they are improving their clinical skills. I know the feeling because I often have it after meeting with Barbara!

Reading through my supervision notes, I can see how Barbara has always been one step ahead of me and able to recognize my patients' main issues from the moment that I present their cases to her. It should come as no surprise that right after the patient described in this chapter left the room for the last time, I immediately emailed Barbara. It was almost as if she had been in the room with me the entire time.

I can see how much I have grown and developed as a clinician since I started working with Barbara. My ability to understand the patient, relate to them, identify patterns, learn about their inner life, and make notes of characteristic issues has allowed me to better support my patients and continue my professional development. I will always be grateful for Barbara's loyalty to the process, her respect and passion for supporting young clinicians, and her ability to improve the lives of patients by supporting me and others. This meaningful relationship is a gift that I will cherish and carry with me for the rest of my personal and professional life.

Notes

1 All identifying information has been disguised to protect the privacy of the client/patient. Any resemblance to actual persons, living or dead, is purely coincidental.
2 Resistance is anything that opposes the work of the treatment. Resistance can also be thought of as a defense, and is an expected element of treatment that helps us understand our patients' characteristic patterns of behavior (Cabaniss et al., 2011).
3 "Enactment" is a pattern of nonverbal unconscious interaction in a therapeutic relationship (Plakun & Erikson, 1998).
4 "Projective identification occurs when one person (A) projects a thought or feeling into another person (B) and then interacts with B to make B experience the projected feeling. We say that in this way, person A maintains an identification with the projected feeling" (Cabaniss et al., 2011, p. 28).

References

Cabaniss, D. L., Cherry, S., Douglas, C. J., & Schwartz, A. R. (2011). *Psychodynamic psychotherapy: A clinical manual.* Wiley.

Plakun, E. M., & Erikson, E. H. (1998). Enactment and the treatment of abuse survivors. *Harvard Review of Psychiatry*, 5(6), 318–325.

Chapter 10

Supervision and the termination process

Anonymous

Preface[1]

The termination phase is an important part of the therapeutic process. It is as meaningful a phase as the beginning and middle parts of treatment. And, like all endings, it is complex, painful, and significant at the same time. Throughout our writing of this book, we kept in touch with an Asian analyst who has been in supervision with Barbara Stimmel since she was an analytic candidate and who continues to work with her remotely today. In this chapter, she writes about how in supervision they worked through her first termination with an analytic patient.

The author asked to remain anonymous to protect her identity as well as the identities of her patients. We are happy to have her contribution mainly because of her unique experience of being supervised on her first termination with an analytic patient. This chapter brings to life the process of termination and the therapist's transition from exposure to the practical theory, to the actual experience of the termination process from the point of view of the supervisee.

Introduction

I began working with Barbara Stimmel when I was a candidate in an analytic training program, where we worked together in person for one year; during this time, I was seeing my patients over Skype. When I returned home, I transitioned back to seeing my patients in person while continuing supervision with Dr. Stimmel over Skype. We would work this way together for another three years.

Supervision gave me a new perspective on the therapeutic work, particularly with difficult patients.[2] Dr. Stimmel helped me understand that analytic listening is a different way of listening entirely, that it is listening to the primary process—the unconscious—and identifying patterns. Sometimes, it was hard for me to listen because I had experienced difficulties working with certain patients. In order to help me, Dr. Stimmel often made associations between my patients' presenting problems and my thoughts about them, which was refreshing and something that I had never experienced in supervision previously. Her hypotheses and formulations about the patients were always helpful. She is very *dynamic* and intuitive; therefore, I was able to recognize my blind spots and think about things in a different way. Despite the cultural and linguistic barriers between us, I always felt comfortable working with her. Ultimately, our work was an integral part of my growth as a clinician.

Culture and language in effective supervision

There is a great cultural difference between Dr. Stimmel and me. I am Asian, and my reserved manner may seem passive or submissive—even obedient. Dr. Stimmel, on the other hand, is very direct, always asking me questions and never accepting "I don't know" as an answer. Her stubbornness and insistence on knowing more details encouraged me to do the same with my patients in order to seek out as much information as I could. I believe that the fact that we were so different made the work with her that much more effective and powerful.

In order to teach me how to be more intuitive in my analytic work, she asked me *not* to prepare written material and discouraged me from taking notes while I was in a session with a patient. Rather, she pushed me to improvise—something that I did not always feel comfortable doing. Nonetheless, I ended up liking it. It took away the pressure of translating every session, four sessions a week, into English. Dr. Stimmel was looking for the nuances that could be found when I was speaking rather than reading. She had always emphasized that there is great meaning in the words the patient uses. In the context of supervision, this was a bit of a challenge because I was analyzing in my native tongue while my supervision sessions were in English. One of the ways we remedied this was by using the chat function during the remote supervision sessions. This allowed me to look up words as we spoke, which decreased my anxiety around not being fully understood. Eventually, I became more comfortable speaking in English, which facilitated the effectiveness of supervision even further.

I appreciated that Dr. Stimmel, because of the idiomatic and idiosyncratic differences between our languages, was curious about how my patients and I communicated during the treatment and if there were changes in the termination phase. A specific and interesting question posed by Dr. Stimmel was if, toward the termination phase, the language became more intimate. I explained to her that no, that with a patient, especially one with whom there is a significant age difference, a certain formality remained. She did not challenge my decision to continue and end the treatment using formal language.

My introduction to termination

I had learned about termination in my studies and throughout my analytic education. In other words, I knew all about termination *theoretically*. However, I had never experienced the termination process with an analytic patient before. Dr. Stimmel introduced the idea of terminating with a specific patient we had been discussing in supervision for over three years. Prior to this, with my non-analytic patients, the treatments were generally shorter, ended more quickly, and to some degree felt much easier.

One day during supervision, as we were discussing this patient, Dr. Stimmel suggested that we think together about what a termination with this patient would look like. I was surprised when the possibility of terminating was introduced. Until then, I had felt very frustrated with this patient and felt that the patient was far from completing treatment. However, my supervisor had a different viewpoint. She reminded me that a lot had in fact been accomplished in the treatment. For example, there was much character change and increased self-awareness and self-reflection. There were also major life changes that the patient had made both in their professional and personal development, including the ability to end a difficult relationship. "The patient is much closer to ending than beginning," Dr. Stimmel would say. In this discussion, she guided me to think about the termination as a *process*, or termination *phase*, and consider the reasons to begin this ending and the benefits it would bring to our work.

Shortly after, I brought up the idea of termination with my patient. We explored it and eventually came to the decision to terminate together. We chose the date on which we would stop treatment, which was ten months from the initial discussion. It helped us understand the significance of establishing an end date. Once we know there is an end date, it is "in the air." It is then that the mourning process can begin.

Despite my initial hesitation, I began to trust myself and trust that the patient had the capacity and ability to terminate. I also learned that the termination process itself was part of the "curative" process because it helped the patient become independent and self-reflective. During the termination phase, in supervision, Dr. Stimmel focused on the relationship between me and the patient. This enhanced the usual analytic attitude of neutrality or abstinence. She tried to teach me how to make the termination more real for the patient and for me. Reflecting back, she may have taken this approach because up until that point in the treatment, the patient had not yet been able to see me as a real person; rather, the patient saw me as an idealized figure.

Throughout the termination phase, the patient became more and more independent and mature. I could see how, at the beginning of the treatment, the patient had looked up to me and idolized me. At the end, the patient appreciated me and our work more realistically—more as a peer, one could say. I felt that my patient and I were now in a different place in our relationship, which was a very powerful realization. We both knew when we would be stopping, and I think this influenced the analysis very much. Before having this experience, I had thought that in order to terminate therapy, the analyst should focus only on character change and symptom relief. While all of that is essential, now my thoughts are a little different. When I start to believe that the patient has developed the ability to think about themselves like an analyst—in other words, to be able to analyze themselves—then that is the time to think about termination.

My growth as an analyst

I had always felt that Dr. Stimmel's opinion of my patients was more positive than my own; but this has been true of all of my previous supervisors. I believed that they were much more hopeful about my patients than I was. They were optimistic about the patient's competencies, and confident that the patient would be able to complete treatment—much more so than I was at the time. At first, I questioned whether it was just my personality that shaped these negative or pessimistic views. My conclusion, however, is that it was not just my personality; rather, it was my limited experience as an analyst.

These days, I feel that I have become much more hopeful about all of my patients. I am able to see more of their positive attributes and strengths. Dr. Stimmel would say that this is connected to my increasing confidence in my own abilities as an analyst. Perhaps because I did not recognize my own potential to learn and grow, I did not hold out much hope for the patient. This is particularly true for the patients whom I viewed as "difficult" or "immature." However, as I would soon learn, I just needed the help of an experienced and confident teacher—someone who believed not only in my patient's ability to do the work but also in my abilities as an analyst. Because my supervisor saw the potential in the patient, it gave me confidence in myself; I did not feel so alone.

One turns to a teacher who is confident—who is not so frightened—in the same way one turns to a doctor for reassurance that everything will be okay. Through the supervisor's confidence in her own ability to teach, the supervisee gains the confidence in her ability to learn; and, ultimately, the patient gains confidence in their own ability to respond. Because my supervisor believed in me, because she saw that I was capable, I was able to internalize this faith and eventually get there myself.

I want the readers to know that a good supervisor should have a lot of knowledge; but at the same time they should also have strong advocacy skills—not just to be there as a listener or provide a different perspective, but to actually act. In my case, Dr. Stimmel had helped me a lot with a problem I had in the institute where I was training. She wrote a letter to the institute and provided some support regarding the continuation of my analytic training while seeing patients via Skype while I was on the Western coast of the United State and my patients were in my home country. Funnily enough, now as we are experiencing the Covid-19 pandemic, online or phone analysis is the only method of work.

The process of termination is a process of mourning. Our patients should be able to look at it head on and say "OK, we are separating." This process is the same between the supervisor and supervisee. I have learned to think as an analyst through the years of working with my supervisor, Dr. Barbara Stimmel.

Notes

1 Preface written by the editors. The author of this chapter wishes to remain anonymous.
2 All identifying information has been disguised to protect the privacy of the client/patient. Any resemblance to actual persons, living or dead, is purely coincidental.

Chapter 11

Supervisor

A daunting privilege

Barbara Stimmel

Preface

Allison Abrams had been my supervisee for a year while a candidate at the Contemporary Freudian Society Psychotherapy Program and, occasionally, I would hear from her with news about developments in her career. Liat Shklarski, who had been in the same training program, was referred for supervision by Allison. Some time later, Allison opened her private practice and asked if we could resume supervision. My work with both women was going swimmingly when one day, during supervision, Liat was very eager to talk about something other than the patient we had been discussing: "Allison and I want to write a book about you as our supervisor; we think we can each write a chapter that would demonstrate how much we have learned and profited from our supervision with you." She went on to present a very thorough and clearly thought out conception of a book about supervision, its benefits, difficulties, learning opportunities, idealizations, disappointments, and much more. They hoped I would give them my blessing, introduce them to some of my supervisees who might be interested in contributing chapters, and write something myself. Liat's and, indirectly, Allison's excitement permeated the room, and I assumed (correctly) that they would not take no for an answer.

Nonetheless, several concerns leapt to mind. First and foremost—how could we recast their creative idea such that its focus was on their central axis rather than on my work as their supervisor? Their premise was that by presenting the work of one supervisor in different supervision relationships, they could demonstrate the power, usefulness, and necessity, really, of supervision in the career-developing, practice-building, and clinical sophistication that is essential in our work, even beyond training requirements. Their strategy of eliminating the endlessly wide variety of supervisory styles, strengths, weaknesses, and so on by using just one supervisor as the fulcrum would more easily and naturally allow the book to achieve those goals. It made good sense; my task then was to help them shift the focus away from me as the supervisor per se, so that the reader would be encouraged to think broadly about the issues rather than dropping in on only one person's work.

A second concern was how to enlist other supervision partners without undue pressure or favor. It became clear that I would make the introduction and Allison and Liat would "do the talking." This is their book, and they needed to be the good editors they have become as they invited, explained, and sometimes convinced my junior colleagues to join in. And this naturally aroused a third concern having to do with my new roles in Allison's and Liat's professional lives. I held being their supervisor in first place, but soon realized that I—or rather, we—had to find a way to easily and productively move among four working dyads as supervisee/supervisor, reader/contributor, compiler/advisor, and editor/assistant editor.

That was asking a lot of us, yet it has turned out to be an extremely rewarding expansion of our work together. None of us has ignored our definitive roles of supervisee and supervisor, but we have gradually and enjoyably incorporated these other ways of thinking and creating together. We began a new project that grew out of our original reason for meeting while also reinforcing the bedrock of our work. Actually, this broadening of our working alliances mirrors that which I will address below, pertaining to the variety of ways in which supervisors and supervisees create professional relationships that extend beyond that of teacher and student.

The final concern I had related to what would be most helpful in the chapter that Allison and Liat had asked me to contribute. I knew that they were inspired to write and edit this book because supervision had become a central element of their increasingly sophisticated and productive professional lives and identities. I had worked with both of them as they opened private practices, navigated all the frame issues of time/fees/insurance/space, etc., dealt with the transferring of patients, and overcame so many of the myriad challenges that present themselves when taking this gigantic step in clinical development. With both women, we continued with supervision as their level of work, decisions, insight, and acumen grew impressively. Their hope to convey to others the importance—or requirement, actually—of ongoing (even if intermittent) supervision throughout this marvelously enlightening and gratifying work was evident in their invitation. I hope I can reinforce their focus on the multiform process of supervision.

Starting out

I would be remiss to write this chapter without starting at the beginning, and that of course is as a supervisee myself. "Supervisee" is an interesting label since it implies that one is a student although also a practitioner. A supervisee sees patients and is responsible for their well-being while also learning how to treat them and help them learn about themselves. Perhaps the most important aspect of being in supervision is that only the supervisee is in the room with the patient, such that the supervisee is required to bring the patient to life in another consulting room—that of the supervisor. This is so obvious that it is often overlooked as the key to unlocking the work of supervision. In this way, a supervisee is learning not only how to work as a therapist but also how to inform the supervisor about what they need most. However, the supervisee is often (certainly in the early days) unaware of what is most important to emphasize, thus the hour is typically filled with a verbatim process to the exclusion of thought and self-reflection. In other words, just like our patients learn how to be patients, supervisees must learn how to be supervisees, how to use the supervisor's expertise, and how to stand outside of their own consulting room to look at the two people within: the patient and them.

I was once such a beginner; I had clinical supervisors, analytic training supervisors, clinical research supervisors, group supervisors, and peer supervisors. I was pretty "supervised-up!" It is no surprise to report that the range of expertise, teaching skills, and clinical subtlety among my supervisors was wide-ranging and diverse. Luckily, I did not cross paths with anyone who was not up to the task and who did not have something to impart that was helpful. But some were a cut above the rest in sharing their clinical knowledge.

My supervisor told me at my first clinic position with my very first patient that, no, I did not have to continue a session with an inebriated client(!). My first analytic training supervisor had never seen a five-times-weekly patient, but there I was with one assigned to me by the referral service—she was very interested in discussing the differences in frequency. Another supervisor encouraged me to write my first paper, and yet another fell asleep during one of our sessions! Group and peer supervisors also had a tremendous impact on my developing skills; they were wonderful, competitive, and supportive—the epitome of good working relationships. My experience as a supervisee was probably just like most of yours in many ways.

I remember how subtly, yet clearly, I learned to imitate, then incorporate, and then identify with those teachers/colleagues as therapists. Although my self-assurance was increasingly enhanced, it took a long while for me to trust that I could be all alone with my patients, even as I allowed my supervisor(s) to leave me more on my own. By this, I mean to describe the realization that I was no longer invoking the words, style, and even presence in my head of my supervisors when working in my own consulting room. In other words, I was developing my own identity and convictions, along with the very important tool of accurate self-assessment. This, which is one of the most important assets of a therapist (or any professional, really), gave me the courage to go forth on my own.

Settling in

The professional path to becoming a supervisor is unfortunately idiosyncratic and unsystematic; my development as a supervisor most certainly reflects that of most of my colleagues. Simply put, I had no specific training beyond the expectation that, as a training analyst/supervisor, I would have had a certain amount of clinical experience. Insofar as supervising the general population of therapists, I was proverbially on my own.

My first supervisee was working at a clinic, and I was very nervous. Could I—would I—rise to the occasion? Was I knowledgeable enough to understand him and his patient? I had a fair amount of experience teaching at college level, but I knew this was very different. I was now expected to impart more than an abstract body of knowledge. I would be asked to share my own clinical understanding of both a patient and his therapist while also teaching technique in a quasi-clinical setting. Since I had no formal preparation for this, I was learning as I went along, and perhaps to some extent at someone else's expense. While on-the-job learning sometimes can be highly effective, and experiencing the "real thing" can be a terrific teacher, it is extremely unwise to ignore the importance of preliminary preparation.

So, in this case, as in many others in life, I called on those who had been my supervisors and served as my models—both positive and negative. Much of this collaboration was outside my immediate awareness as I was fortified by identification. But sometimes, even if clumsily, I quite deliberately used their language, styles, and words of wisdom. Thus, slowly but surely, I integrated the two, and, in the process, I developed my own self as a supervisor. Although it was daunting, it was also exhilarating! And ironically, but not surprisingly, this of course mirrored my behavior as a supervisee. But then, is that not the way in all educational endeavors?

Hearkening back to my supervisor who had never conducted a five-times-weekly analysis, when I presented with a patient ready to come in at that frequency, I watched an outstanding clinician and teacher learn from her student. She was frank about her curiosity and even her envy, a bit. I learned not only critically important first steps in starting an analysis, but also how to question important ideal versions of analysis. My supervisor was an honest and sharing partner in our work as we helped the patient ease into the role of analysand, and she helped me begin to sense that I could do this work. She proved that the most important lesson when teaching is the imperative of learning from those we teach.

Some years ago, I had a wonderful corollary opportunity to examine this complex issue of learning, teaching, and teaching how to teach when I was asked to chair a new sub-committee on supervision for the Committee on Psychoanalytic Education (COPE) of the American Psychoanalytic Association (APsaA). Our committee learned much over the decade or so that we met. After carrying out a national survey, we discovered that hardly any institute in APsaA, including several American institutes independent of APsaA, offered seminars, experiential learning opportunities, or even reading lists to supplement and support the development of supervisory skills. In other words, no one was being formally taught how to be an educator.

There is an old saw in medicine, "see one, do one, teach one." Unfortunately, that legacy from the medical imprint on training in America has left our profession without enough formal education in becoming an educator; not none, but certainly not enough. In the interest, and hope, of making a dent in that serious omission, our committee developed a reading list for the website and began an ongoing course at the bi-annual meetings of APsaA with invited speakers at each forum. We held an ongoing discussion group for many years on supervision; the room was always filled with beginning clinicians, residents, graduate students, analytic candidates, seasoned clinicians, and training analysts from around the world. We all want to learn from each other because that is the most profound pathway to increased skill and self-awareness as a clinician. Needless to say, we learned so much when doing that work—more than just what was needed in the more formal education of supervisors and increasingly how one might teach supervision. Teaching teachers takes a special skill because one is also indirectly teaching the teachers' students. And although our course had just gotten off the ground when APsaA's administrative structure changed, it is my expectation that the focus on this extremely central part of training remains strong.

This experience dovetails nicely with another fortunate ongoing experience in my work as a supervisor in which, in addition to my supervision of an analyst's own caseload, I often turn to their work as a teacher of supervision. As a result, I supervise at least two tiers of a supervisee's work as a therapist and as a supervisor. And in this way, I am reminded very directly of how much opportunity there is for modeling in the supervisory relationship. We are repeatedly asked to impart many forms of knowledge—clinical, intellectual, theoretic, practice-building, and frame-setting knowledge—along with opening and closing the door to our patients. Teaching how to teach is among the most rewarding mutual learning experiences in my clinical day. Despite not being in formal training, some of my supervisees are doing private supervision and will occasionally ask for help in developing an understanding of doing this work in addition to receiving supervision of their clinical work. As suggested above, this is one of the ways that the supervisor and supervisee extend their working relationship as the teacher/student pair becomes a pair of working colleagues.

This shift in the dynamic of a given supervision dyad brings to mind one of the most important issues in any educational relationship: the cultural variance between student and teacher. I have taught, supervised, and evaluated colleagues from around the world to become training analysts, but I have particularly worked with colleagues from Korea and China.[1] There are genuinely important cultural differences that must be recognized so that critical listening, understanding, and exchange can take place. It goes without saying that it is imperative for a clinician in this context to learn and comprehend these differences in order to be more sensitive to nuance and perspective. Supervisors, interestingly, must be especially sensitive to these demands because they do not have the luxury of experiencing the same free association, dreams, and intimate revelations that help clinicians learn about so many of the less obvious aspects of their patients' lives.

Engaging in supervision with my Asian colleagues has been an enriching and very special aspect of my professional life. The many ancillary joys inherent in looking at the world and my work through a very different lens have added to the great pleasure of teaching. Yet, in ways for which I was not initially prepared, I came to understand the importance of knowing as much as I could about almost all aspects of their national traits, customs, language, food, etc. A clinical kaleidoscope was placed in my lap.

For example, the fact that Korean people take off their shoes upon entering homes meant that I needed to let go of my automatic focus on the clinical meaning of a patient's removal of his shoes when lying on the couch. Straightforward, yes, but it is still clinically interesting because there are layers of meaning in what one wears inside their shoes! Koreans have two languages, formal and informal, such that the subtleties of change in a patient's productions eluded me for a long while—they do not use first names, do not know their exact birthdays, and celebrate the Chinese New Year. And then, despite sharing broad Asian customs, there are endless discoveries to be made about daily life in China that make it different from life in Korea, and certainly different from life in the United States.

The following experience had a tremendous impact on my understanding of the supervisory relationships between me and my Korean supervisees. When conducting a seminar with Korean colleagues, I was completely unprepared for the rigid hierarchical structure to which all students and their teachers were expected to conform: members of the student audience could only ask questions in order of seniority among them, it was considered rude to ask questions directly, and the idea that a lecturer could be wrong was unfathomable. I worked very hard on trying to position myself so that I remained respectful of their customs while also encouraging a possible softening of these regulations. My own teaching was delimited by their lack of spontaneity or participation, which is so essential to and invigorating in an American educational setting. As implied above, we had a culture clash! But we all worked hard at moving closer to each other's position, and thus to each other; in the process, we all learned a great deal that went far beyond psychoanalysis.

In this way, I gained a different perspective on how my supervisees from halfway around the world experienced me in my role as a teacher and in their role as students. Some of them were senior psychiatrists in their hospitals and medical schools, but when placed in the role of student, they accepted the lower social stratum that came with it. I had to learn what my position was in the hierarchy while quietly but persistently trying to minimize this divide between us. Some supervisees still will not call me by my first name, but I am convinced that they too have worked hard to understand our cultural differences so that they can accommodate me. Yet the cultural divide persists, runs deep, challenges understanding, and in this way is another layer on top of that which forms the centerpiece of our work: "truly" knowing one another. Who said psychoanalysis and psychotherapy were easy?

This anecdote is apposite because it captures how critically important it is to remain open to all voices in the room, whether many or one. It is critically important to bend and flex outside of one's comfort zone; it is critically important to learn and change on the proverbial spot. This is an apt description of good supervision. The implicit "cultural" differences pertain to experience, self-confidence, years of practice, and yes, authority and hierarchy. These last two are unavoidable but neither automatically destructive nor dangerous.

When referring to authority, I mean the ability to influence others because of one's recognized knowledge about something. When referring to hierarchy, I mean the arrangement of people such that they are considered above, below, or at the same level with regard to their knowledge alone—this is not a reflection of their innate ability, goodness, or intelligence. Supervisors are probably too often assigned indiscriminate hierarchical authority by their supervisees. It is therefore incumbent upon the supervisor to be wise, judicious, open, honest, sharing, complimentary, and, most important, generative. The better supervisors are sensitive to this complex context so that they can steer their students toward a more even playing field, one on which both teams can win.

Yet it is not surprising, and perhaps it is even more pleasurable than broadening my cultural horizons, that I have come to appreciate, again, the universal substrate of the human condition through supervision. This commonality does not eliminate all these differences that appear among us—it simply allows us to recognize and respect them ever more deeply. Also, cross-cultural differences highlight the demand that we recognize and respect those differences that are closer to home. Of course, I am referring to differences in gender, sexual orientation, age, religion, ethnicity, training, professional grouping, etc. Without simplifying this dizzying array of demarcation, I simply aver that the necessary and concomitant ability to stand in someone else's shoes is the sine qua non of good therapeutic and supervisory relationships.

A long time ago, one of my first patients, a New York City Police Department detective, challenged me to go on a "ride along" in a police cruiser so I could get some idea of his daily life; otherwise, how could I ever hope to help him? I felt on shaky ground, not knowing a thing about being a police officer, but as he challenged me, I realized that I did not know a thing about many other professions either; nor did I know anything about being French/Italian/Israeli/Latvian/Japanese, Catholic, Black, southern, old, gay, male … the list was obviously endless. Nonetheless, I also did know something, actually many things, about all of those categories and any others one could name, including that of NYPD detective! The hope is that education, intelligence, curiosity, empathy, and insight—all in the service of a commitment to care—can help soften the edges of difference and ignorance. Our shared humanity also allows us to transcend divergence while fostering common roots. This is not to ignore the insurmountable limitations imposed on us by our irreducible subjectivity. Nonetheless, these borders are sometimes permeable, making possible good—or even excellent—psychoanalysis and psychotherapy, and allowing for good—or even excellent—supervision.

Expanding horizons

As the world shrinks, our professional reach extends. Distance learning has become a mainstay in our work as institutes conduct classes, lectures, and seminars over the telephone and computer. Clinicians have followed suit with teletherapy and telesupervision. I have been taking this approach to my supervision with foreign supervisees for a while. In some instances, I have met and worked with a supervisee first in their home country and then worked with them remotely from my office in New York; with others, we first began in New York and continued online after their return to their respective countries. In some other arrangements, we have yet to meet in person. My former assessment was that the telephone and computer are simple, non-determinative elements in supervision. However, I learned from work closer to home that this was not the case as a virus set the stage for potential enactment.

New York City went on pause—or, more accurately, the city shut down in the spring of 2020 in response to the global Covid-19 pandemic. Those supervisees with whom I had only worked in my office moved to telephone supervision as we seamlessly picked up from our previous in-person meetings. Clearly, one of the great advantages of using technology is that it increased my sensitivity to the experience between the therapist and the patient when they were on the phone or computer.[2] But in focusing on that, I ignored another piece of the puzzle having to do with what was going on between *us* as the supervisor and supervisee, so that, after some time, two supervisees began to find telesupervision wearying. They reported independently that it was increasingly difficult to find anything of value to discuss. As I gave this more thought during the shared and frightening reality that engulfed the world and particularly heavily my home, New York City, it became apparent that something else was happening. This reflection helped me refocus on a central thread in all supervision relationships—the inherent therapeutic tapestry that runs through it.

It is important here to underscore my insistence that supervision is not therapy. Precisely because the supervisor is a teacher and not a therapist, the supervisor needs to maintain boundaries so that slippery slopes are avoided. Nonetheless, parallel processes abound, and all players are susceptible to their enticing pull.[3] Unusual settings and stresses can easily strengthen that pull in ways that are unexpected and yet unsurprising. A proverbial blind spot disrupted my vigilance to the constant undercurrent of the "therapeutic" component of supervision as I was working with my supervisees in my own city via telesupervision.

The telephone (and computer) seem to offer intimacy such that it may seem two people are together while actually far apart, each in their own private space. The advent of the telephone allowed people to be together in ways never before imagined while simultaneously creating the exact opposite experience as well. This phenomenon is beautifully described by the poet Proust on the telephone for the first time:

> "Granny!" I cried to her, "Granny!" and would have kissed her, but I had beside me only that voice, a phantom, as impalpable as that which would come perhaps to revisit me when my grandmother was dead.
>
> (Proust, 1952, p. 129)

It was time for me to pay attention to that phone and all that it may have surreptitiously invited into our work. My supervisees, along with everyone else, were struggling with social isolation, and yet here they were, pseudo-close with a therapist whom they trusted. Their complaints about supervision were very likely not just due to "tele-fatigue"[4] but also related to other feelings that had been stirred up that they wished they could discuss. Having nothing to talk about may very well have been a classic reversal of how much they wished to speak about other things. I do not know if I was correct in this assessment, but recognizing that this was occurring (even if it was not in the forefront of their minds) helped me to help them focus on what we were doing and why.

And that speaks to the broader point. Although clinical insight is often not that far out of reach, it is best to stay in the role of teacher while safeguarding against being drawn into that of a therapist in interactions with supervisees. Although there are "therapeutic" moments in all relationships, especially when being understood in new ways, I remain adamant that supervision and therapy are entirely different undertakings. Since others may disagree, I will expand on my particular way of working in this regard.

To begin, I adhere to the insistent principle that supervision is not therapy for the sake of the supervisee, whose privacy is of the utmost importance; this speaks for itself. Although second on this list, the safeguarding of our patients is constantly kept at the forefront. My concern is that when one brings to bear the role of clinician in supervision, the inverse is also likely; that of supervising when conducting therapy. This worry is less about what one might say and more about what one might hear, as it were. Listening is always colored by expectations, regardless of how agenda-less one is. Since most patients are not students of analysis or therapy, our role as a supervisor might seem a distant danger. However, we know that patients come looking, and sometimes even begging, for answers. In response, a central precept of our work is to help our patients increase their personal agency so that they are disabused of the longing for others to make choices for them, offer dictates, and provide paths for them to follow. Thus, the therapist must create strong fortifications against the teacher/student dynamic that is implicit in all therapy.

Finally, as the supervisor engages in an enactment, there is an implicit invitation for the therapist to do so with the patient. While that in itself is to be guarded against for the therapist's sake, the ultimate loser is the patient the supervision dyad is discussing. It stands to reason that not only obvious mistakes and omissions will occur in supervision but that, in this instance, a whole other, unidentified "presence" enters the room. This likely and unfortunate possibility can occur due to the therapist's susceptibility to importing the parallel process into the therapy. The unavoidable and threatening triangulation that appears in supervision is to be expected. Being sensitive, unafraid, and, equally important, unashamed of these enactments are the supervisor's best instruments of instruction. Particularly because these scenarios are part and parcel of our work as clinicians, we must expect them to play out in supervision—how could they not?

The narrative of a primary transference illusion, that the therapeutic dyad is an inseparable whole, is in part ironically created by the reliability of the physical boundaries that exist ethically in the therapeutic relationship. Wishes safely will not come true. Thus, perhaps in telesupervision, the safety implicit in the distance between supervisor and supervisee ironically strengthens the attraction of the therapeutic undertow, and then, why not in both directions?

And here my insistence on a therapeutic frame of only in-person meetings invited me to ignore that which was in front of me (most likely all along) with my supervisees around the world. Therefore, although we do not analyze, interpret, or work in the transference in the teaching relationship, its frame is certainly (at least in part) built on the safety, support, and even love akin to that in the therapeutic one.

Just as we expect that therapy and supervision share some felicitous features, we must also be on the alert for the myriad mazes that abide in both sets of dyads. I am of course referring here to resistance to the work and the supervisor's assistance, the splitting of the transference between the supervisee's therapist and supervisor, and that most insidious difficulty, idealization, and its soulmate, derogation. As banal as this may be, it is imperative that we expect, and accept, less-than-hoped-for outcomes, difficult interactions, and outright failures. How could I not have missed the boat with some, disappointed others, and met those whom I knew I could not and perhaps did not want to reach? All couples need chemistry to cohere, and the supervision dyad is no different; the "fit" is fundamental.

Moving on

I hope it has become clear that supervising is one of the most rewarding parts of my professional identity and of my day. When thinking about the purpose of this book and what I could add to help demonstrate the key role that supervision plays in all of our work, it made sense for me to situate my approach within my theoretical/clinical orientation. What I hope I have shown is that, regardless of one's own predilections, one's dedication to teaching should be powerful enough to overcome any differences. If it is possible to do that (as described above) within the context of personal and cultural differences, it seems likely that we can supervise without imposing our own theoretical "culture" on our supervisees as well.

This seems a good place to "confess" that I am a thorough-going classical Freudian psychoanalyst; or, as some might say, a dinosaur! Most of my practice has been the four- or five-times-weekly psychoanalysis of adults. I also completed child analytic training and have spent some years working with children and their families. Serendipity played a role in my having developed a steady presence of couples in my practice as I have recognized the effectiveness of an analytic perspective in helping couples identify and appreciate the more subtle dynamics that prevail in all relationships. And finally, I did research on sexual dysfunctions in a hospital setting so that I have also seen over the years people with explicit difficulties with whom I work within a behavioral model. In other words, although my core identity is that of a classical analyst, my daily work is a tapestry woven with many threads. I listen to all things through a classical prism, but I live and work in a very wide world of models, colleagues, and patients. It is safe to say that although my "third ear" is bent in a certain direction, it is attuned to a variety of vibrations.

An interesting example of this possibility is found in my supervision with a Lacanian-analyzed and trained therapist. We began our work in the traditional institute setting of a more-or-less classical orientation. We rarely encountered differences in technique since the classroom and ambient atmosphere dominated. We focused on the patients presented in this way, and our work together was rewarding. After a period of time, the supervisee decided to return to her clinical roots while at the same time asking me to come along. We were both aware that this could be an unusually productive exchange or it could end dismally. A Freudian and a Lacanian listening to the same patient with one "teaching" the other?! It is of course important to remember that Lacan was a deeply knowledgeable and proud disciple of Freud, even as he developed quite divergent therapeutic techniques—chief among them the "arbitrary" ending of the session.

Our decision to go ahead was not that different in the end than any other confrontation with cultural roadblocks in teaching and treating, and what we discovered was not a surprise: form (technique) follows function (analysis). Since we were devoted to the same function, the variety in our forms was interesting, mutually informative, and therapeutically productive. All three of us—the patient, the therapist, and the supervisor—benefitted and grew. If one listens in a particular direction but uses an array of attunements, the possibilities of therapeutic and educational success are wide and deep.

Ending

I am not truly at the end, but rather continuing to engage in this work that I love and that helps define me. What I have written about here has hopefully described my choices across many aspects of my being. As I am nearer to the closing than to the beginning of my professional life, it makes sense to reflect on the whole of it thus far to serve as a natural conclusion to this chapter.

The supervisory relationship, like other relationships in life, requires watering, feeding, questioning, and answering. It cannot exist with only one participant; therefore, it demands cooperation and trust. While it is easy to wax poetic about two people struggling with this very demanding work of psychotherapy, it is also quite quotidian. This is not an insult; rather, it is a very fair and encouraging description because the everyday is not only familiar but also masterable, learnable, graspable, and understandable. The most successful supervisors not only love teaching, they love mastering, learning, grasping, and understanding, too.

I think the most important takeaway from all these years that I have spent supervising is recognizing that saying "I'm not certain, I will think this through and have more to say next time" is among the most honest and meaningful sentences a supervisor can utter. It seems that, as a model, it demonstrates the humility that is critical in the best caretakers; as an admission, it reflects the truth that no one person knows everything; and, as an invitation to revisit the question, it opens the door for true collegiality. Simply put, the best supervisors keep their own supervisor models close, demonstrate their willingness to share, constantly refuse to dictate interventions, and, perhaps most importantly, allow those they are educating to find their own ways—even as they surpass them. When we think about it, that is really the ethos to which we aspire as analysts and therapists.

Thus, as practitioners, through our own particular prisms, we help those on our consulting room couches and chairs work through their obstacles to trust, intimacy, and pleasure. The most profound assistance we can offer is in easing the tension between the persistent human desire for closeness and the inexorable march throughout life toward separation and loss. Proust eloquently penned this as a description and metaphor when thinking of his beloved grandmother. One description of "growing up" is in tolerating the transformative loss that accompanies every figurative step forward. Good analysis, therapy, and supervision help bring about the essential sublimation that describes maturity.

Finally, it is important to note (as this book underscores so well) that asking for another ear to listen to a case that presents vexing clinical problems is central to achieving our best work. Years of meaningful and ongoing informal mutual supervision with my analyst friend made our weekly lunches more nourishing than the food on the plate; I cannot imagine any seasoned clinician not turning to a colleague for "supervision." I know that it is what separates the clinical wheat from the chaff. Good luck as you join me.

Notes

1 As a member of the Board of the International Psychoanalytic Association (IPA), I had the privilege of working with the Korean Study Group; and, as faculty and a supervisor, I worked with the China American Psychoanalytic Alliance (CAPA).

2 I do not conduct therapy sessions over the phone or computer as I have insistently resisted the lure to enable easy access and not cancelling sessions, etc. Yet, many (most?) therapists have become comfortable and proficient in this way of working. But for me, it has always made (and still does make) eminent clinical sense to be together in

the same room at the same time, while avoiding the additional resistance it produces. However, disease and disaster have required that I loosen some of my convictions, adapt, and learn; like everyone else, I now use the telephone to treat. When I return to my office, the telephone will resume functioning solely as a tool for patients to leave me messages, but for now, I am a convert—writing as I am during a pandemic.

3 In an earlier paper, I described an enlightening experience as a supervisor that captured the possibilities of working through resistance to a "blind spot" that allowed for the felicitous outcome of the eye-opening(!) advancement in our work (Stimmel, 1995).

4 A term I coined to capture the common complaint among at-home workers; it is exhausting.

References

Proust, M. (1952). *The Guermantes way* (C. K. Scott Moncrieff, Trans.). Modern Library.

Stimmel, B. (1995). Resistance to awareness of the supervisor's transferences with special reference to the parallel process. *International Journal of Psychoanalysis*, 76, 609–618.

Index

Figures are indexed in italic page numbering. Tables in bold page numbering